DAHN
YOGA
BASICS

DAHN YOGA EDUCATION

Healing Society

6560 Highway 179 Ste.114

Sedona, AZ 86351

www.hspub.com

928-204-1106

Copyright © 2006 by Dahn Yoga Education

All rights reserved. No part of this book may be reproduced or transmitted in any form or by any means, electronic or mechanical, including photocopying, recording, or by any information storage and retrieval system, without permission in writing from the publisher. For information, address Healing Society, Inc., 6560 Highway 179 Ste.114, Sedona, AZ 86351.

First paperback edition: November 2006

Library of Congress Control Number: 2006931388

ISBN-13: 978-1-932843-17-0

ISBN-10: 1-932843-17-5

Manufactured in China

If you are unable to order this book from your local book seller, you may order through www.amazon.com or www.hspub.com.

A COMPLETE GUIDE TO THE MERIDIAN STRETCHING,
BREATHING EXERCISES, ENERGY WORK, RELAXATION, AND
MEDITATION TECHNIQUES OF DAHN YOGA

DAHN YOGA BASICS

DAHN YOGA EDUCATION

Healing Society

My body is not me, but mine.

My mind is not me, but mine.

I am the master of my mind and body.

—Ilchi Lee

How to Use this Book

This book is organized according to the four comprehensive stages that comprise the Dahn Yoga training method.

The first component of Dahn Yoga training is Meridian Stretching. Used primarily as preparation for more intense training activities, it loosens up the upper body and strengthens the lower body.

The second step is Jung-Choong Breathing, which combines sequential movements with focused breathing. This practice facilitates energy accumulation and proper energy circulation.

The third training category is DahnMuDo, which combines Dahn principles and traditional Korean healing martial arts to enhance mental and physical strength. Through the discipline required of this practice, personal character and integrity are also enhanced.

The last and fourth stage of Dahn Yoga involves meditative energy work. At this stage, practitioners learn to achieve great stillness of mind while increasing sensitivity to the movement and flow of Ki energy. This practice eventually progresses to vision meditation, which allows participants to re-create their lives as they most desire by infusing the mind with positive thoughts, feelings, and imagery.

Any of these four steps can be an effective training method when done independently. However, the best results are achieved when all four steps are practiced daily as a one to one-and-a-half hour training session.

Note: Always listen to your body. There is no need to rush your progress and push through your discomfort. All bodies are unique, and you will find your own level of practice naturally. If you are on medication that makes you drowsy, foggy, or hyperactive, please consult your health professional before beginning practice.

Foreword

"My body is not me, but mine."

This is a phrase that Dahn Yoga practitioners around the world speak with great enthusiasm. Its meaning has been central to the Dahn Yoga method since its beginnings in a small Korean park in the early 1980s. As the practice has developed over the last 25 years into a global training method, this phrase has continued to be an essential element in Dahn training.

The training techniques of Dahn Yoga are designed to develop mastership of the body and mind through the medium of energy, which is the means of communication between the body and mind. Through this process, one comes to understand experientially the true meaning of "My body is not me, but mine." Once this level of mastership has been achieved, one may apply this experience to the full spectrum of everyday life.

Since I created Dahnhak (the original name of Dahn Yoga) based on traditional Korean mind-body training methods, the basic philosophy and principles of Dahnhak have not changed, but the training methods have been continuously revised and improved.

As humanity's understanding of the human body has increased, many people have tried to create an easier and more effective training system based on the teaching experiences of Dahn Yoga instructors and their students. This book is the result of those efforts.

One of the most simple and effective concepts in Dahn Yoga is the idea of "breath." All living beings breathe. It is necessary for survival on this planet. However, it is taken for granted by most people. Few people pay attention to their breathing. But the quality of the breath has great implications for the health of our mind and body.

Whether people pay attention to their breath or choose to ignore it, they will continue to inhale and exhale. Through the experiential understanding of the breath achieved in Dahn training, the connection between mind-body communication and the breath becomes more apparent.

Breath also dramatically demonstrates the interconnectedness between people. The air and energy that one person breathes in is also the same air and energy other people have just breathed in and out. Awareness that everyone shares the same air cultivates the understanding that all living things are interconnected, not only through the breath but on many levels. Ultimately, this understanding helps develop more caring, open-hearted individuals and in turn creates a more harmonious world.

Imagine that a bell sits on the floor in front of you. No matter how great the bell is, if you don't ring it, there is no sound. The same is true with Dahn Yoga. Dahn Yoga is not a theory, but a practical way of life. Include Dahn Yoga as part of your daily practice and stick with it so you can experience its full benefit. I sincerely hope that this book will help you take your first steps toward a healthier, happier, and more peaceful life.

ILCHI LEE
Founder of Dahn Yoga

Contents

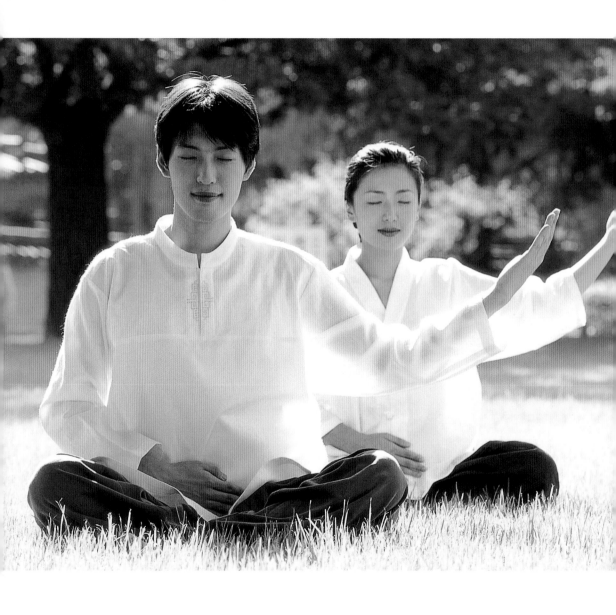

PART 1

WHY DAHN YOGA?

Straighten your body, and stand tall in the world. Those who have no shame in their minds straighten their bodies and are always composed.

—*Cham-jun-kye-kyung* (ancient Korean sacred text)

What Is Dahn Yoga?

Dahn Yoga is an integrated mind-body training method that combines deep stretching exercises, meditative breathing techniques, and energy awareness training. Its objective is to help practitioners achieve their highest level of personal potential.

The traditional name for Dahn Yoga is "Dahnhak," which literally means "the study of energy." In Korean, "Dahn" refers to the primal, vital energy which is essential to all life forms, and "Hak" refers to the study of a particular theory or philosophy. Thus, a Dahnhak practitioner is one who studies the system of energy for the purpose of personal self-development.

During Dahn Yoga training, practitioners learn to communicate with their bodies through energy. As the body's energy circulation is stimulated, its innate natural healing power is activated. Through consistent practice, practitioners can lead themselves back to optimum health. Essentially, they regain true mastership over their bodies through the medium of energy (Ki).

The benefits of Dahn Yoga, however, extend well beyond physical health. For one thing, the concept of "health" is all encompassing in Dahn Yoga. A truly healthy person not only has a fit and functioning body, but also seeks balance and harmony in all areas of life. Practitioners of Dahn Yoga often report that through their practice, their family life improves, they gain confidence in their career, and many old and burdensome emotions are finally released.

When practitioners arrive at their goal of a healthy life, they often extend their intentions by creating harmonious relationships with their family, friends, communities, and nature. This helps them to become better human beings and creates a healthier, happier, and more peaceful world.

What Are the Benefits?

Dahn Yoga was created for people who want to live better lives and gain flexibility and balance of body and mind, even while living their busy, hectic lives. One of the advantages of Dahn Yoga is that it is easy and simple enough for anyone to learn, yet challenging for even the most advanced practitioner. Anyone – male or female, young or old – can enjoy the various programs and benefits of Dahn Yoga. Regular practice can offer you the following benefits:

FOR YOUR BODY The combination of breathing techniques and deep stretching movements evenly work every muscle and joint in your body to:

- Increase flexibility and balance.
- Improve respiration, energy, and vitality.
- Improve bone density and muscle tone.
- Help maintain a balanced metabolism.
- Promote cardio and circulatory health.
- Help manage pain in the body.
- Increase circulation to all organs of the body.

FOR YOUR MIND All postures in Dahn Yoga are designed to unify movement, breathing, and awareness. This is what makes Dahn Yoga different from ordinary stretching. Paying careful attention to proper posture while controlling your breathing and concentrating completely on the here and now can:

- Help you relax and handle stressful situations more easily.
- Teach you how to quiet the mind and concentrate well.
- Encourage positive thoughts and self-acceptance.
- Create centeredness and balance.

FOR YOUR SPIRIT Dahn Yoga can be used purely to promote physical and mental well-being. However, this system is comprehensive, integrating not only the physical and mental, but also the spiritual aspect of human existence. Dahn Yoga practice helps you develop a peaceful mind and stimulates your spirit to:

- Become aware of your body, your feelings, and the world around you.
- Help you feel whole and connected with humanity and nature.
- Help you find your life purpose and rekindle your passion for life.

How Is Dahn Yoga Different?

Dahn Yoga is similar to other forms of mind-body training, but it can be distinguished by three unique characteristics:

THE MASTERY AND USE OF ENERGY Energy is a defining element in Dahn Yoga because it is considered to be the medium that unites body and mind. Practitioners develop a deeper understanding of their bodies through energy while experiencing directly the connection between mind and body and strengthening communication between the two.

From the perspective of energy, Dahn Yoga is made up of five stages: initiating, accumulating, controlling, commanding, and completing. Practitioners first learn how to feel and accumulate energy in the major energy centers of the body. As the sense of energy gradually develops, formerly blocked energy channels open up, promoting circulation of energy throughout the body. Once able to control and command energy, practitioners experience natural healing in their bodies while gaining control of emotions and habits.

It is possible to follow Dahn Yoga training without feeling energy. However, when practitioners feel energy, they experience the true character of Dahn Yoga and, more than anything else, the training itself becomes more joyful and grows into a multidimensional experience.

ENHANCING THE BODY-BRAIN CONNECTION Dahn Yoga contends that the brain is not simply an organ, but is, in fact, the center of the whole human body and its energy system. Through the various Dahn Yoga programs, practitioners can learn to utilize their brain fully toward the creation of a better life for themselves and those around them. However, the power of the brain is not limited to individual and personal development. Just as the human brain can create strife and intolerance in the world, so too can it create a peaceful, healthy society.

SELF-MANAGED, HOLISTIC HEALTH CARE The Dahn Yoga program includes principles and techniques for improving emotional patterns, as well as physical condition. In particular, it has many elements that improve the quality of social interaction and communication skills. It is also helpful for correcting unhealthy habits, such as smoking, overeating, and the like. As will be explained in greater detail later, the key principles of Dahn Yoga and its systematic methods of training make this possible.

Where Did It All Begin?

The roots of the Dahn Yoga extend several thousand years back into Korean history. It began as a training program designed to educate the Korean population for the development of both mind and body. It was practiced on a daily basis with the intention of maintaining people's health and developing their potential to become ideal humans. Up until 2,000 years ago, this educational method was practiced and transmitted by wise men to each generation. Dahnhak contributed to the health and political unity of the Korean people for many hundreds of years. However, the Korean people failed to keep the Dahnhak tradition alive.

During his personal journey toward self-realization and self-discipline, Ilchi Lee rediscovered the tradition and modernized it. He first started teaching Dahnhak to a stroke patient he met in a small park in Anyang, Korea. In 1985, the first Dahn center opened in Seoul, Korea. Since that time, the program has expanded throughout the world with more than 600 centers offering Dahn Yoga to more than 200,000 active practitioners. The tradition of offering the exercises continues in thousands of public parks, schools, assisted living centers, and college campuses in Korea, the United States, Canada, Japan, and other countries.

Getting Started

LOCATION   No specific location is necessary for Dahn Yoga training. It can be practiced indoors or outdoors. The training methods introduced here can be used in your office or at a rest stop when you need a break during a long road trip. To enjoy the maximum benefits of Dahn Yoga, however, it's good to have a set place for your practice. Choose a quiet location with little noise and enough space for stretching. Also, make sure that the temperature is neither too hot, nor too cold.

CLOTHING   Wear comfortable attire that does not inhibit movement. We recommend clothes made of a natural fiber that are absorbent, lightweight, and breathable. It's a good idea to train without shoes, if possible.

TRAINING TIME   It is best to train two to three hours after eating. Dahn training includes movements that bend the body forward or backward and twist it from side to side, so you might feel discomfort if you train on a full stomach. Training in the morning is a great way to kick off an energy-filled day, but you should choose whatever time works best for you.

Try to set a fixed time for training, if possible—ideally, one to one-and-a-half hours. However, if this is not practical, you should train for at least 20 minutes. It is best to train every day, but if this is not possible, then two to three times a week is sufficient. Although this book will serve as a basic guide, the best way to learn Dahn Yoga is to get the instruction and guidance of a professional instructor at a Dahn center.

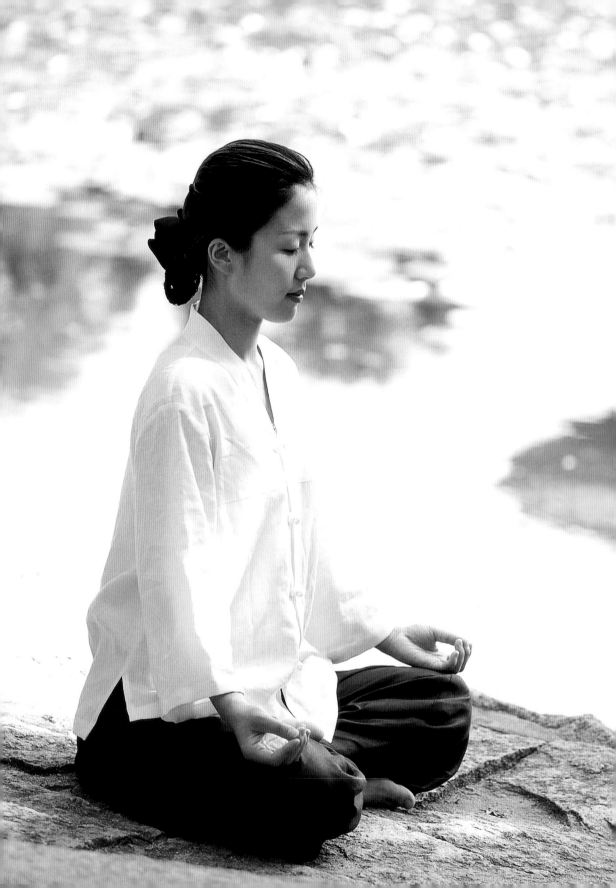

PART 2

UNDERSTANDING
THE BASICS

In our minds resides the bright light of divinity ever driving us to seek the same brightness that, once enlightened unto us, makes us realize that Heaven, Earth, and Human are all One.

      —*Chun-bu-kyung* (ancient Korean sacred text)

Energy System of the Body

Ki, the Life Energy

Ki, also commonly spelled Chi or Qi, is a fundamental concept embraced by Asian philosophy, arts, medicine, and mind-body traditions. *Ki* is the word for the vital energy that is the true essence of every creation in the cosmos. Most people begin their understanding of Ki by experiencing it as bio-energy, or the basic life force in the body.

Ki is the bridge linking the body and mind; it is the essence of life, moving and flowing freely. The continuous joining together and drifting apart of Ki comprises the rhythm of the phenomenon of life. Everything in existence undergoes constant change. Everything around us, as well as our very lives, are temporary manifestations of Ki.

Although immersed in this grand flow of energy every moment of our lives, we are unable to sense its currents without properly attuned senses. Our overdependence on rational thought and language has obscured our natural ability to sense the flow of energy. However, we can regain our innate ability to feel the slight but pervasive vibrations that define our existence. It is up to us to reawaken this "sixth sense." By opening blockages in the energy pathways and reawakening our innate ability to sense energy flow, we can recover our health and natural balance. When we develop sensitivity to Ki, we will be able to utilize our bodies' potential more fully.

Energy of the Mind, Jin-ki

There are three types of Ki energy in the human body. *Won-ki* is the energy that you have inherited, or were born with. *Jung-ki* is the energy that you obtain by eating and breathing. And *Jin-ki* is generated through deep, concentrated breathing. Won-ki and Jung-ki are generated without conscious participation, while Jin-ki requires concentration. The energy that is utilized in Dahn Yoga is this Jin-ki.

Since Jin-ki is generated by the mind through concentration, its quality varies according to the state of the mind at a given time. A positive frame of mind and emotional state produces a positive flow of energy. This, in turn, will have a calming and relaxing effect on the body. A negative state of mind and emotions will have the opposite effect. When the flow of Jin-ki is blocked or impeded, the body becomes tense, resulting in stagnant energy.

We often use the concepts of Chun-ji-ki-woon and Chun-ji-ma-eum in Dahn Yoga practice. Chun-ji-ki-woon is another name for cosmic energy. In Korean, it means the highest level of Ki that circulates throughout the universe. We experience Chun-ji-ki-woon when we have Chun-ji-ma-eum, which means Cosmic Mind or "Enlightened Consciousness."

Energy Channels and Energy Points

The meridian system is a series of channels which transport Ki through the body. Meridians can be compared to a system of irrigation canals carrying sustenance to the body, mind, and spirit. Acupressure points, which are distributed along the meridians, are energy ports through which energy enters and exits the body.

Imagine that the meridians are the paths for the transport and supply of goods. If you see the body as representing land, the meridians represent the main highways, while the acupressure points can be viewed as bus stops and resting places. Just as one may transport goods following the roads, your body can supply energy to the organs and different parts of the body through meridians. If energy flows well through the meridians, it is distributed evenly through the body, helping both the body and the brain to maintain their optimal condition.

Your body consists of 12 major meridians and eight minor meridians. In general, only 14 of the meridians are commonly used. Ki comes into the body

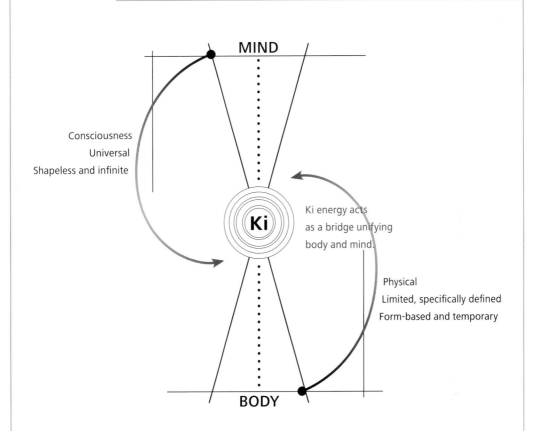

MIND

Consciousness
Universal
Shapeless and infinite

Ki

Ki energy acts
as a bridge unifying
body and mind.

Physical
Limited, specifically defined
Form-based and temporary

BODY

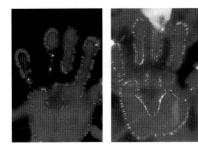

The Kirilian energy photo
on the left shows a hand
in a normal state. The picture
on the right shows the same hand
emitting Ki.

through the breath. It then flows through the 12 meridians and collects in two of the eight extra meridians—one along the back, called the Governing Meridian (Dok-maek), and one along the front, called the Conception Meridian (Im-maek). The two meet when the lips touch.

Each of the 12 major meridians is associated with one of the principle internal organs and is named accordingly: kidneys, liver, spleen, heart, lungs, pericardium, bladder, gall bladder, stomach, small and large intestines, and the triple burner (body temperature regulator). Yin meridians flow upwards. Yang meridians flow downwards. These 12 meridians are paired, or bilateral, and situated systematically on either side of the body. Ki flows constantly through the 12 meridians of the body, starting with the lungs and ending in the liver.

Important Energy Points

These are the energy points most important in Dahn Yoga training. Becoming familiar with them will prove very beneficial for you.

BAEK-HOE: Located at top of the head, it lies at the intersection of an imaginary line that connects the ears and a line that connects spine and nose. "Baek-hoe" literally means "intersecting point of 100 meridians." This is the point where energy flows in.

JUN-JUNG: Located about four to five centimeters in front of the Baek-hoe, this is also a point where energy flows in. While Baek-hoe is sometimes called "Great Heaven's Gate," Jun-jung is named "Small Heaven's Gate."

IN-DANG: Frequently called "the third eye" in the West, this point is located between the eyebrows. When this point is activated, one might exhibit extra-sensory perceptual powers.

MI-GAN: Located at the top of your nose, in the center of the indention at the top of the blade of the nose.

IN-JOONG: Located in the center of the valley between your nose and lips.

AH-MOON: Located between the first and second vertebrae. This is the place where the neck and head meet.

OK-CHIM: Locate the slightly protruding point in the back of your head. Ok-chim consists of two separate points that are located one inch to either side of that protrusion.

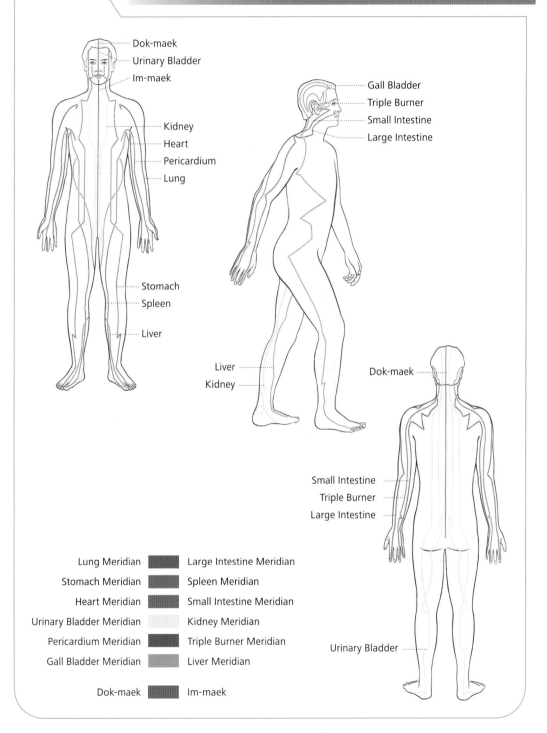

Dok-maek
Urinary Bladder
Im-maek

Kidney
Heart
Pericardium
Lung

Stomach
Spleen

Liver

Gall Bladder
Triple Burner
Small Intestine
Large Intestine

Liver
Kidney

Dok-maek

Small Intestine
Triple Burner
Large Intestine

Urinary Bladder

Lung Meridian — Large Intestine Meridian
Stomach Meridian — Spleen Meridian
Heart Meridian — Small Intestine Meridian
Urinary Bladder Meridian — Kidney Meridian
Pericardium Meridian — Triple Burner Meridian
Gall Bladder Meridian — Liver Meridian

Dok-maek — Im-maek

TAE-YANG: Located on the temples, in between the eyes and the tops of the ears, these are important activation points related to the brain.

DAE-CHU: Located right below the seventh cervical vertebrae.

DAHN-JOONG: Located in the center of the slight indentation on the chest.

KI-HAE: Two inches below the navel. Ki-hae means "the sea of Ki-energy." The lower Dahn-jon is located about two inches inside the body from the Ki-hae.

HOE-EUM: The perineum.

MYUNG-MOON: Located on the back, directly opposite the navel, between the second and third lumber vertebrae. "Myung-moon" means "the gate of life." Cosmic vital energy enters the body through this point during Dahn-jon breathing exercise.

JANG-SHIM: Located at the center of the palm on each hand. To find the Jang-shim, make a fist. The point is where the middle finger touches the palm. Because it is very sensitive to energy, it is viewed as an external Dahn-jon energy center.

YONG-CHUN: To find the Yong-chun, divide the main body of the foot into three equal parts. Yong-chun is one-third the distance from the top of the toes at the center of the sole.

Key Energy Centers (Dahn-jons)

Directly translated, the word Dahn-jon means "field of energy." It is the main place in the body where energy is gathered and stored. With enough energy sensitivity training, we can tangibly feel the gathering of energy in the Dahn-jon. Basically, Dahn-jon has the same meaning as the word "chakra," which means "wheel or circle" in Sanskrit and is considered an energy center in the human body.

In Dahn Yoga, we focus on three internal Dahn-jons and four external Dahn-jons. The internal Dahn-jons are located in the lower abdomen about two inches from the navel (lower Dahn-jon), in the middle of the chest (middle Dahn-jon), and in the center of the forehead (upper Dahn-jon). The four external Dahn-jons are located on each palm and on the bottom of each foot.

If a Dahn-jon is blocked and energy flow is disrupted, it will manifest as a physical disease or ailment. Through exercises and breath work, it is possible to facilitate the flow of energy through the Dahn-jon system of the body,

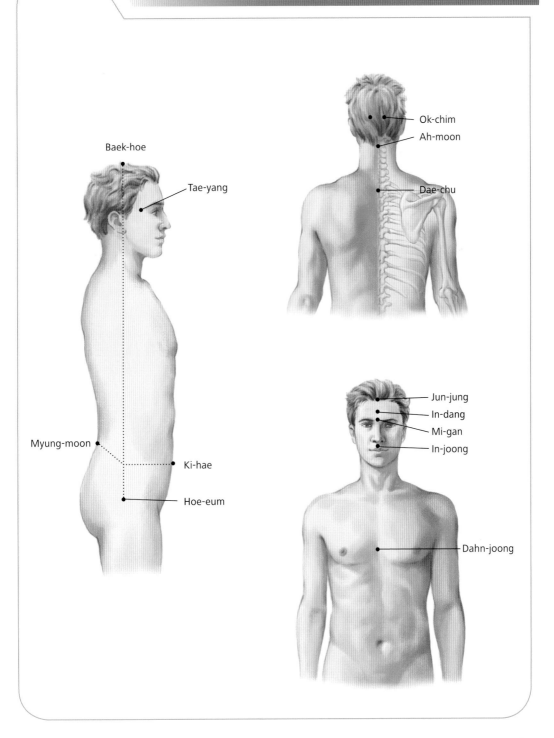

Baek-hoe

Tae-yang

Ok-chim

Ah-moon

Dae-chu

Myung-moon

Ki-hae

Hoe-eum

Jun-jung

In-dang

Mi-gan

In-joong

Dahn-joong

resulting in overall balance and health.

The three internal Dahn-jons are defined by the roles they play. The lower Dahn-jon acts as the fuel tank in which energy is stored for circulation throughout the body. When your lower Dahn-jon becomes strengthened, the overall energy balance of your body will be restored, amplifying your natural healing power. You will exhibit more patience and drive, developing a stronger sense of self-confidence. Red is the symbolic color of the lower Dahn-jon.

The middle Dahn-jon is associated with control of the energy. It is located at the exact center of the chest, between the breasts. Because emotional energy is controlled at this point, strengthening of the middle Dahn-jon will impart a peaceful and loving feeling. Blockage of the middle Dahn-jon, which can occur due to negative emotions and stress, can have an undesirable effect on the nervous system, leading to many different diseases. The color of the middle Dahn-jon is gold.

The upper Dahn-jon is equated with the spiritual aspect of our existence. When the upper Dahn-jon is strengthened, our spiritual ability awakens and we feel a connection with the divine energy of the cosmos. Blue violet is the symbolic color of the upper Dahn-jon.

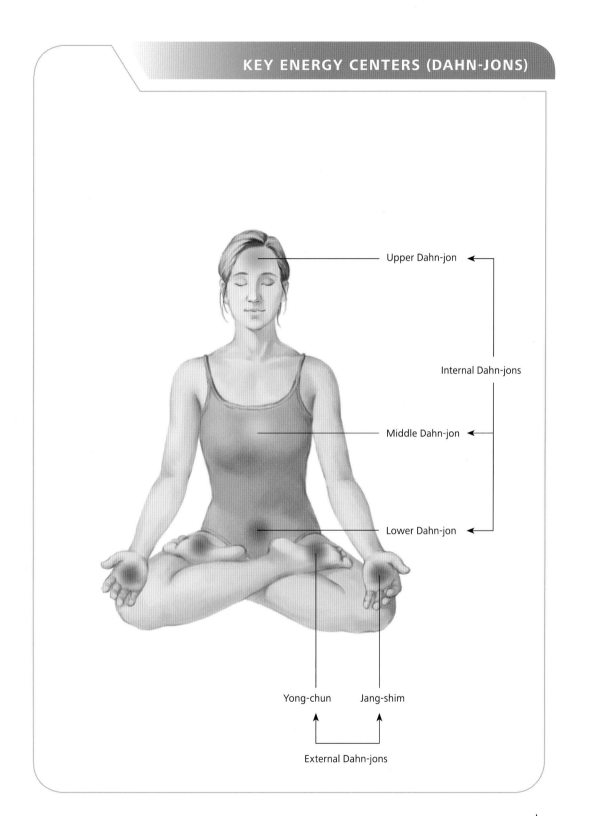

Upper Dahn-jon

Internal Dahn-jons

Middle Dahn-jon

Lower Dahn-jon

Yong-chun   Jang-shim

External Dahn-jons

Through breathing in and breathing out, we drink in Heaven; through food, we eat the Earth. These beings who stand magnificently between Heaven and Earth, endlessly creating, are humans.

—Ilchi Lee

The Dahn Yoga Principles

Su-seung-hwa-gang

Cool water energy and hot fire energy flow within our bodies simultaneously. When the body is in balance, the cool water energy travels upward toward the head while the hot fire energy flows down to the lower abdomen, where it is stored. The underlying principle behind this natural flow of energy is called Su-seung-hwa-gang (Water Up, Fire Down).

We can readily observe examples of Su-seung-hwa-gang in the natural world. Think about the cycle of water on earth. When the fire energy of the sun shines down on the earth, the water energy of rivers, lakes, and oceans rises to form clouds.

Consider how plants obtain their energy. They receive fire energy from the sun shining down on their leaves, while drawing the water energy up through their roots from moisture in the ground. With this cycle of energy, plants and trees grow and bear fruit. In the winter, when the ground is too frozen for plants to draw up water, leaves fall to the ground and no fruit is produced. Life itself goes into dormancy until the natural cycle of energy is once again possible.

Su-seung-hwa-gang is the core principle for human health. When the human body is in balance, the cool water energy travels upward toward the head along the back side of the body, while the hot fire energy flows down the front side of the body to the lower abdomen. This constitutes a complete cycle of energy circulation. By repeating this circulation, life maintains its balance and continuity. Perhaps you have heard the expressions: "I have a fire in my belly" or "Keep a cool head."

The kidneys and the heart facilitate this natural circulation with the help of the body's energy center. The kidneys generate water energy in the human body while the heart generates fire energy. When the energy flow is smooth and balanced, the Dahn-jon imparts heat to the kidneys and sends the water energy up. This cools the brain and brings down the heat from the heart so that fire energy moves downward.

When the water energy travels upward along the spine, the brain feels cool and refreshed. When the fire energy flows down from the chest, the lower abdomen and intestines become warm and flexible. In this cycle of energy flow, the Dahn-jon, the energy center in the lower abdomen, performs the most crucial function.

If the energy flow is reversed and fire energy moves upward while water energy moves downward, then the abdomen may be clammy and the neck and shoulders feel stiff. You may feel "weak at heart" or fatigued. In this state, many people experience problems with digestion, including chronic constipation, tenderness in the lower abdomen, and circulatory problems.

There are two common reasons for improper action of Su-seung-hwa-gang. The first occurs when the Dahn-jon, which acts to draw in and store energy, is too weak or inefficient to do its job properly. In this case, the mind becomes cluttered with incessant thought as fire energy moves upward to the brain.

Stress can also interrupt Su-seung-hwa-gang because it negatively affects the downward flow of energy through the chest. When this flow is blocked, energy backs up and returns to the head, resulting in anxiety and nervousness.

When "Water Up, Fire Down" is in effect, your lower abdomen is warm while your head is cool. Your hands and feet are warm, and you have plenty of saliva in your mouth. You can perceive with greater clarity of mind and your senses are opened. You feel positive and relaxed, and your creativity and imagination are enhanced.

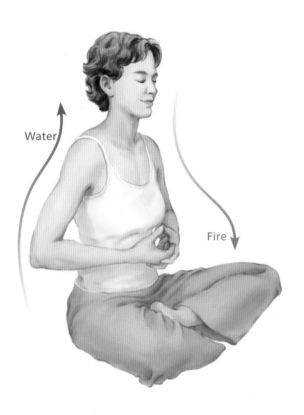

Water

Fire

Water Up, Fire Down (Healthy State)	Fire Up, Water Down (Unhealthy State)
Circulation, dynamic, lively	Disconnected, static, lifeless
Sweet saliva in the mouth	Dry mouth, bitter taste
Warm hands and feet	Cold hands and feet
Cool and refreshed head	Heat and pain in the head
Warm abdomen filled with energy	Abdomen lacks warmth and energy
Regular bowel movements	Constipation, digestive problems
Refreshed and energized	Tired and uncomfortable

Jung-choong, Ki-jang, and Shin-myung

Jung-choong, Ki-jang, and Shin-myung means, "The body is filled with energy, our energy becomes strong, and our spirituality is awakened." These three terms are collectively referred to as the Sam-bo, which literally means the "three treasures" of the human body. Jung-choong, Ki-jang, and Shin-myung refer to the process of energy control and maturation. This principle emphasizes the fulfillment of the lower Dahn-jon, the physical energy center, as the basis of the development of the entire energy system. This can be explained by a comparison to construction. Without a stable and strong foundation, you cannot build up to high levels.

JUNG-CHOONG: THE BODY IS FILLED WITH ENERGY

Jung, the physical body, is the vessel of earthly life that you have received from your parents. The physical body is sustained with breathing and eating. The lower Dahn-jon, associated with the physical body, is completed when it is filled with Jung energy derived from food and breath. When you have reached the level of Jung-choong (Jung fulfilled), then you have achieved optimal physical condition through the completion of the lower Dahn-jon. Increased adaptability to new surroundings and resistance to disease will result. When your Jung is "fulfilled," then you will experience the truth of "My body is not me, but mine." You will be able to control your sexual energy and channel it according to your will.

KI-JANG: ENERGY BECOMES STRONG

Ki, the energy body, is strongly influenced by mental and emotional energy, which emanates from the middle Dahn-jon. For the Ki to become strong or mature, your heart must open to receive the natural wellspring of love and peace within. Strengthening of the Ki allows control of emotional energy according to your will. In other words, you will realize that your emotions and your thoughts are not you, but yours to command.

SHIN-MYUNG: SPIRITUALITY IS AWAKENED

Shin-myung represents the completion of the upper Dahn-jon. At this stage, your consciousness exists with an elevated sense of awareness, accomplishing total integration of the physical, energy, and spiritual bodies while imparting

THE STATE OF JUNG-CHOONG, KI-JANG, AND SHIN-MYUNG

Shin-myung

Completion of the upper Dahn-jon
Enlightenment and spiritual development
Confidence, insight, and totality of being

Ki-jang

Completion of the middle Dahn-jon
Mature love, joy, and a sense of peace
Wholeness, compassion, and empathy

Jung-choong

Completion of the lower Dahn-jon
Optimal physical condition
Enhanced life force

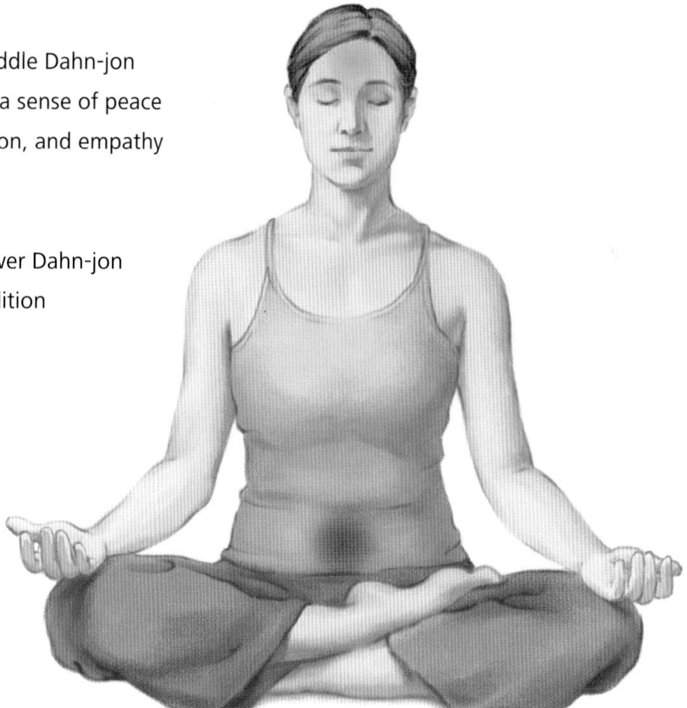

a sense of purpose to life. You will develop superior insight and judgment, frequently "knowing" the underlying principle of matter without a conscious learning process. You will manifest consistent creativity and develop an overriding desire to create harmony and order in all that you see.

Shim-ki-hyul-jung

The principle of Shim (Mind)-ki (Energy)-hyul (Blood)-jung (Body) states: "Where consciousness lies, energy flows, bringing blood and transforming the body." This phrase implies that consciousness is the true reality behind the appearance of form. A simpler way of saying Shim-ki-hyul-jung is, "Energy goes where mind goes." Try this simple exercise to experience Shim-ki-hyul-jung.

Breathe in and out a few times to relax your whole body. Concentrate intently on the center of your palms. Keep concentrating and imagine that your palms are becoming hotter than the rest of your body. After a while, if you measure relative temperatures with a thermometer, the temperature of your palms will have increased compared to the rest of your body. This phenomenon occurs because your conscious concentration sent energy to your palms, increasing circulation and warmth.

When you develop deeper sensitivity, you gain the ability to send energy to any part of your body. You can warm or cool a specific part, if you so desire. With an amazing switch located deep within your consciousness, you can draw on the infinite energy of the cosmos at will. With enhanced concentration comes increased ability to control this access to energy.

When you align consciousness, energy, and body with one single wish and have developed the strength and maturity to maintain and protect that single wish, you will recognize the amazing power of your mind. You will witness the wish, a thought in your consciousness, come into being in the world of form. You will have become a creator in the fullest sense of the word.

To clarify your understanding of Shim-ki-hyul-jung, imagine using a magnifying glass to gather and focus sunlight. If you move the glass around instead of leaving it in one place, then the sunlight will scatter. However, if you maintain exact focus in one place for a prolonged period of time, then the sunlight becomes strong and enough heat builds to create fire. Our thoughts are similarly powerful, capable of generating concentrated energy to express our own divine creativity.

The principle of Shim-ki-hyul-jung provides fundamental guidance for the process of evolution, creation, and the existence of all things. When consciousness becomes concentrated, energy starts to gather. This in turn begins to attract the material necessary to manifest the essence of the concentrated consciousness. Hyul, which literally means "blood," actually refers to all the material required to generate the shape and form of a wish. Therefore, Shim-ki-hyul-jung refers to the process of the invisible consciousness creating a tangible form through the power of concentration.

This is why every sage in the history of humankind has told us to be careful with our mind and our thoughts. An unconscious wish is still a wish and an unconscious curse is still a curse. It is crucial to be continuously aware of what we think and how we act and speak. We must also develop the discipline and the will needed to align our words and actions with our wishes. The universe is filled with information and energy that we can draw on to manifest our innermost dreams and visions…whatever they may be.

When the heart is pierced deeply by an earnest desire to seek the Truth, the mind empties itself, and the infinite life of the cosmos reveals and realizes itself through us.

—Ilchi Lee

Signs of Healing

Jin-dong: The Vibration of Life

For practitioners, fundamental changes occur in the body during the exercises. The changes differ from one person to the next. Without some understanding of what is happening to the body as a result of the Ki stimulation, some people might feel frightened or confused when they experience Jin-dong.

One sign that the body is changing is when the body begins to shake. This reaction is the result of a person moving into a deeply relaxed, alpha brainwave state. As a person begins to feel the flow of energy circulating throughout the body, the body will often shake violently as blockages in the meridian channels are cleared by the new flood of energy. Jin-dong can best be compared to suddenly opening a water faucet connected to a garden hose. With the increase in water pressure, the hose begins to shake violently. Likewise, the body will vibrate when energy suddenly begins to flow.

There are two types of Jin-dong. In one case, Jin-dong occurs when a sufficient accumulation of energy is reached and it begins to flow rapidly through the meridian system. In another case, Jin-dong can result from an influx of vital cosmic energy after fully opening the mind.

Practitioners with good energy circulation may not experience Jin-dong at first. But, eventually, every practitioner experiences Jin-dong, the vibration of life. In other cases, practitioners may not know that they are experiencing Jin-dong because the vibration is so delicate. When individuals persist with the practice and certain parts of the body are revitalized, even healthy people can experience Jin-dong.

Jin-dong can be experienced as a continuous vibration for a certain period of time. It will eventually begin to weaken and eventually completely stop. When practitioners experience Jin-dong, there is a temptation to become preoccupied with the phenomena. However, spending too much time absorbed in the phenomena will exhaust anyone.

Jin-dong can be controlled consciously since it is related to being in a state of relaxation from the lowering of brainwaves. Jin-dong is a sign that Dahn Yoga practice is reaching a plateau, and a person's health will improve after such an experience. After experiencing Jin-dong, most people feel refreshed since the blocked meridian channels have been opened. The mind feels steady and strong, and physical health improves dramatically.

Myung-hyun: Alternating Brightness and Darkness

Nature is cyclical. Day turns to night, and night turns to day. The body's energy system is also a climate, continuously fluctuating between dark and light. Dahn Yoga exercises increase and free energy, making it lighter and brighter as heavier energy is released. In the process, toxins held by stagnant energy are washed out of the body.

As the energy system begins to release stagnant energies, numerous uncomfortable sensations, called Myung-hyun, may appear. Myung-hyun literally translates as "brightness" (myung) and "darkness" (hyun). The symptoms persist until energy is able to flow freely. Although Myung-hyun may feel uncomfortable, its symptoms indicate that the body is restoring itself. The Myung-hyun phenomena may include both physical and emotional symptoms.

Practitioners may feel unexplained levels of fatigue or experience flu-like symptoms. After the symptoms disappear, energy levels increase. Bruise-like stains can appear on the skin at the sites of old injuries, or an old pain may return for a short time. Similarly, practitioners may experience a recurrence of a health problem or an unusual physical sensation, such as a persistent vibration in some area of the body. Strong waves of cold or heat could suddenly emanate from the center of the body. These symptoms indicate that healing has started to occur at the energy level, rather than just at a physiological level. Physical Myung-hyun symptoms are alleviated when the basic energy flow of the body is optimized to the state of Su-sueng-hwa-gang.

Myung-hyun phenomena can also occur when an individual's old emotional habits begin to change and negative emotional energies are released. Emotional Myung-hyun can manifest as inexplicable mood swings, sudden depression, or angry outbursts.

Remain positive and grateful for the opportunity to become more energetic. Where your mind goes, energy follows. If your mind is bright and positive, bright and positive energy will come to you.

If you experience Myung-hyun, you may not want to continue your practice. However, maintaining your practice is usually the most efficient way to recover. If you go to a Dahn Yoga Center, consult your instructor.

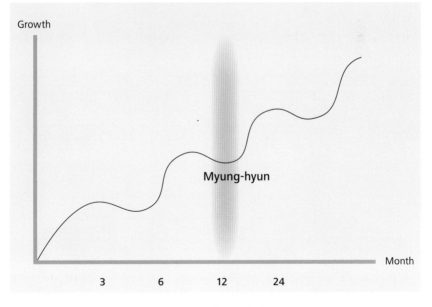

[Progress of practice]

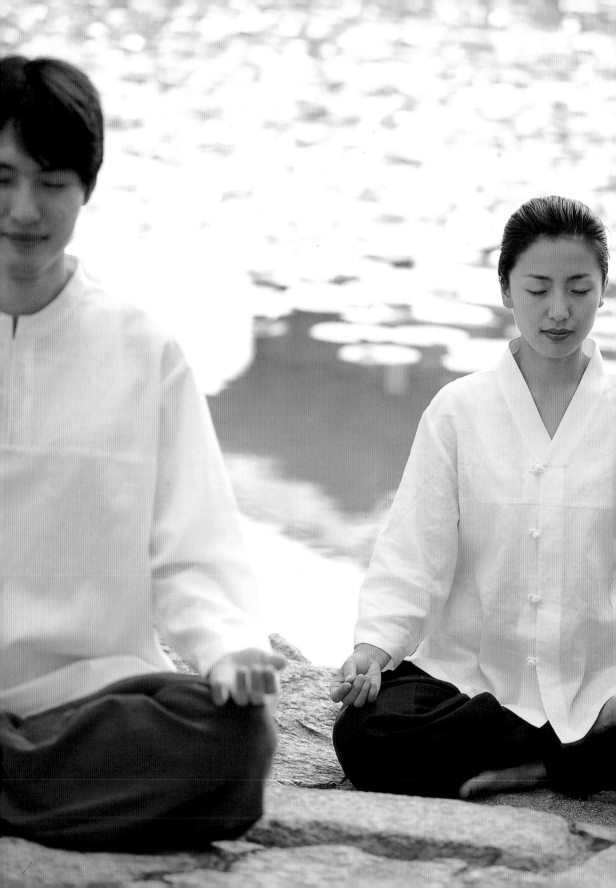

PART 3

DAHN YOGA IN PRACTICE

To take another breath, we must first exhale. When we have breathed out and emptied our lungs, we can breathe in again.

—Ilchi Lee

The Components of Dahn Yoga

The Dahn Yoga program consists of four main components based on the previously-mentioned principles of Jung-choong, Ki-jang, and Shin-myung. These four components can each be an effective training method when done independently. But the best results are achievable if all are performed together over a one to one-and-a-half hour daily training session.

Meridian Stretching (for Preparation)

These are warm-up exercises to prepare the body for collecting energy. There are hundreds of Meridian Stretching exercises. In this book, however, we are only introducing the most effective movements for helping the body collect energy. These movements relax the upper body and let the center of the energy come down into the lower Dahn-jon. They also focus on limbering up the pelvis, which is like a bowl that collects the energy, and the hip joints, which are like energy faucets. Meridian Stretching is also utilized as cool down and finishing exercise.

Jung-Choong Breathing (for Jung-choong)

A set of breathing postures designed to restore the Su-seung-hwa-gang state to the body, Jung-Choong Breathing helps to build energy in the lower Dahn-jon and unblocks the body's two main meridians. Consistent practice of these postures will improve energy accumulation and circulation in the body and stimulate the body's natural healing ability.

DahnMuDo (for Ki-jang)

DahnMuDo is the combination of Dahn principles and Korean Traditional Healing Martial Arts. Through the practice of DahnMuDo, we can master the method of moving and spreading energy accumulated in the Dahn-jon through the whole body. In this non-combative, healing martial art, we learn how to use our body to enhance our mental and spiritual strength while gaining a sense of personal integrity.

Relaxation and Meditation (For Shin-myung)

In Dahn Yoga, practitioners focus on energy to create the meditative state. They usually begin by focusing on energy between the palms. While increased sensitivity to energy is a definite benefit of this practice, it is not the end goal. Rather, the goal is to help calm an individual's thoughts and emotions, which are the root cause of the stress held in the body. As the sensation of energy increases, the body and mind become more and more relaxed. In this stage, practitioners learn to re-create their lives through vision meditation, which infuses the mind with positive thoughts, feelings, and imagery.

Component	Purpose
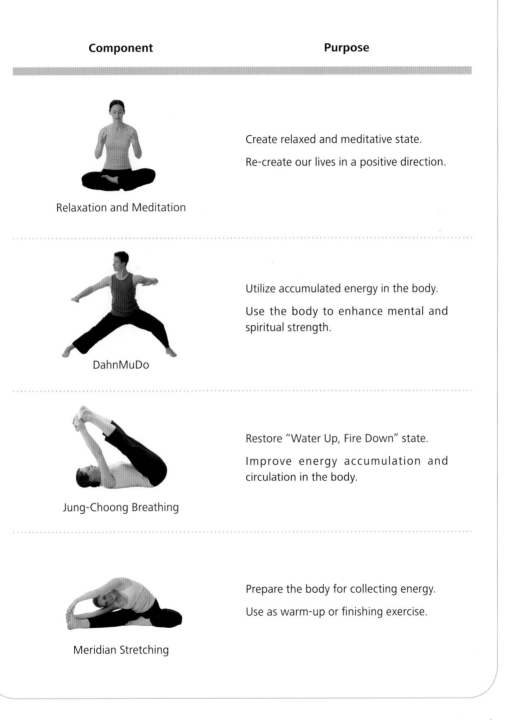Relaxation and Meditation	Create relaxed and meditative state. Re-create our lives in a positive direction.
DahnMuDo	Utilize accumulated energy in the body. Use the body to enhance mental and spiritual strength.
Jung-Choong Breathing	Restore "Water Up, Fire Down" state. Improve energy accumulation and circulation in the body.
Meridian Stretching	Prepare the body for collecting energy. Use as warm-up or finishing exercise.

The person with a safe center doesn't fear change. We can choose change
without fear before a challenge only when we are strongly centered.
—Ilchi Lee

Meridian Stretching

Meridian Stretching is designed to open the meridians of the body and to balance the energy of their associated organs. Meridian Stretching combines proper breathing with stretching movements. When breath is combined with body movement, metabolism can be influenced more effectively.

When the circulation of energy and blood is blocked and stagnant, the Ki sensation becomes dull. Before the beginning of main training, Meridian Stretching revives Ki sensation, which is the core foundation of Dahn Yoga. It helps smooth out energy circulation by eliminating stagnant energy in the body, relaxing the body, and supplying rejuvenated energy. Although used primarily before and after main training, practicing Meridian Stretching on its own greatly helps to maintain health and to prevent illness.

Relaxing the Upper Body

Breathing and meditation cannot be fully experienced when tension is held in the upper body. When the shoulders and chest are blocked in this way, energy stagnates in the upper body, rather than in the Dahn-jon. If the body is not relaxed enough during breathing and meditation practice, the healthy state of Su-seung-hwa-gang can be reversed, rather than corrected. Therefore, Meridian Stretching focuses on relaxing the upper body by drawing the energy down into the lower Dahn-jon.

The Basic Posture

This is the basic posture for all Meridian Stretching exercises in the standing position:

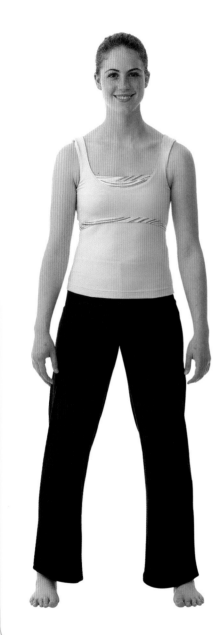

SHOULDERS Relax the shoulders.

WAIST Straighten the waist and curl up the tailbone inward, like a hook. When curling up the tailbone, the S-curve of the spine is straightened and a gentle strain is present in the lower abdomen.

KNEES Bend the knees slightly and naturally. Avoid locking the knees since this can block energy flow.

LEGS Spread your legs shoulder-width apart. Spreading them too wide can scatter the energy of the Dahn-jon and lower body.

FEET Position the feet parallel to each other, in the shape of the number 11. Spread them no more than shoulder width to avoid losing Dahn-jon energy.

SOLES Balance your body weight evenly on both soles.

BREATHING When stretching, focus your mind on the area where you feel tension. Inhale gently through the nose, imagining healing energy flowing to that part of your body. Open the mouth slightly, exhale naturally, and feel the blockage releasing from your body.

Making the Hip Joints Nimble

Meridian Stretching includes various movements to make the hip joints flexible and strong. This is necessary because each hip joint acts as a faucet for collecting energy into the lower Dahn-jon. Training the muscles around the hip joints makes the circulation of energy and blood flow smoother while helping the accumulated energy in the Dahn-jon move and spread throughout the body.

Harmonizing Movement, Breathing, and Awareness

In order to optimize the effects of Meridian Stretching, movement, breathing, and awareness must be harmonized. Start the movements while inhaling. Hold your breath for a moment while holding the posture and then exhale slowly while returning to the beginning position. The body should be centered at the lower Dahn-jon and your consciousness should be focused on the areas being stretched during the movements. When exhaling, imagine that the impure, stagnating energy in the body is leaving with every exhalation. With the mind, imagine that you are having a conversation with the body and focus on the changes or sensations occurring in the body.

It is important to practice Meridian Stretching in a way that is suitable for your body. For example, a healthy person can train more intensely, whereas a weaker person could practice the movement much more gently. Even ill and very fragile people can benefit from gently rubbing and massaging the whole body while breathing and focusing on the consciousness. In the beginning, try to master the movements first rather than attempting to harmonize the breathing and movements. Practice the movements according to your breathing capacity (without straining) when you are familiar with the movements.

BODY BOUNCE

Benefits: This exercise will help you reduce tension and stagnant energy from your whole body. It enhances blood and Ki circulation and relaxes the body.

Note: Breathe naturally and comfortably while rhythmically bouncing the entire body up and down.

1. Stand with the legs shoulder-width apart.
2. Bend the knees slightly and begin to bounce gently.
3. Rhythmically bounce the entire body up and down. Sweep the sides of your body with your fingertips as you bounce.
4. Turn the body 45 degrees to the left and rhythmically bounce the entire body up and down.
5. Turn the body 45 degrees to the right side and rhythmically bounce the entire body up and down.

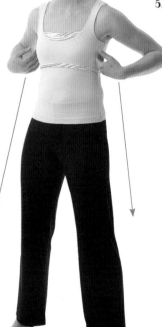

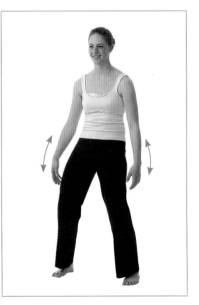

UPPER BODY TAPPING

Benefits: This exercise will help circulation, open blockages, and release stagnant energy from your whole body. It enhances blood and Ki circulation and relaxes the abdominal area.

Note: If you feel discomfort in any area of the body you are tapping, do so more lightly. This is particularly important if you experience stomach distress. Also, do not press into that area. Instead, gently rub hands together and lightly massage that area.

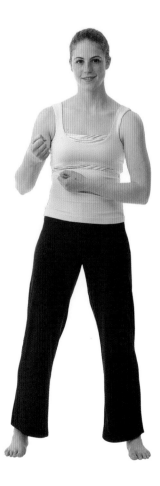

1. Relax the upper body, bend your knees slightly, and balance your weight evenly on both feet.
2. Make a light fist and gently tap the chest, the stomach, ribs, and whole abdomen area while exhaling with a "Aaah–" sound.
3. Continue this motion for five minutes.
4. Focus your consciousness on the areas where you feel achy and stiff, then breathe out with the feeling of letting out the impure energy accumulated in those areas.
5. Close your eyes and focus on the vibration of the tapping as it penetrates deep inside the body.

MERIDIAN STRETCHING

WHOLE BODY PATTING

Benefits: This is a very effective method to reduce tension and release energy from your whole body. By patting, cells are strengthened as they are stimulated and energy points are opened.

Note: Pat the body gently and comfortably to achieve the desired results. You can concentrate better if you allow your eyes to follow your movements.

MERIDIAN STRETCHING

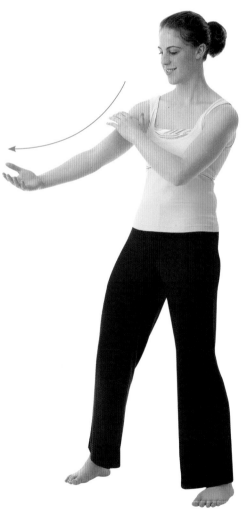

1. Curl your fingers and lightly tap all over your head and face with your fingertips.
2. Stretch out your left arm with your palm facing up. Take your right hand and, starting at the left shoulder, pat rhythmically downward all the way to the left hand.
3. Then turn your left hand over and, with your right hand, pat your way back up to the left shoulder again.
4. Repeat Step 2 and Step 3 with the left hand and right arm.

5. Pat your chest with both hands several times, breathing deeply and exhaling completely.

6. Starting from your chest, pat your ribs, abdomen, and sides.

7. With both hands, pat the area just below the right rib cage where your liver is located and concentrate on radiating positive, clear energy to the liver.

8. With both hands, pat the area just below the left rib cage where your stomach is located and concentrate on bringing healing energy to your stomach.

9. Bend over slightly from the waist and pat the area on your lower back (on both sides) where your kidneys are located and move up, patting as far as your hands can reach. Then pat your way down to your buttocks.

10. Starting from your buttocks, pat your way down the back of your legs to your ankles.

11. From the ankles, start patting your way up the front of your legs until you reach your thighs.

12. From your upper thighs, pat your way down the outsides of your legs to your ankles.

13. From the ankles, pat your way up the insides of your legs to your upper thighs.

14. Finish by striking your lower abdomen about 20 times. This exercise is most effective when done with the legs shoulder-width apart with the knees slightly bent.

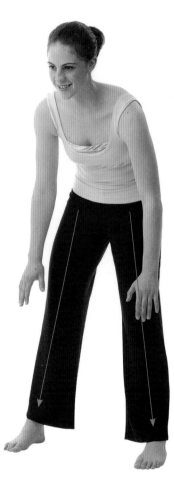

NECK STRETCH

Benefits: This stretch eases tension, increases flexibility, and tones the neck muscles. If your neck starts to feel tight in the middle of the working day, this is a simple way to release the muscles.

Note: Maintain focus on your neck as you perform these movements. Move only your neck and head very slowly. Relax the rest of your body.

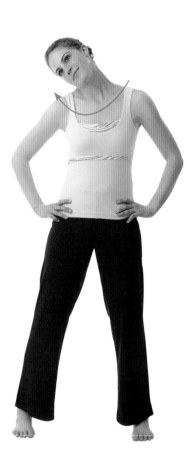

1. With hands on your waist, breath in and push your chin slowly down to the chest. Exhale and return.
2. Inhale and stretch your neck backward. Feel your chin stretch. Exhale and return.
3. Breathe in and bend the head sideways to the left, trying to touch the left ear to the shoulder.
4. Repeat the movement in the opposite direction.
5. Breathe in and slowly turn your head to the left. Exhale and return.
6. Repeat the movement in the opposite direction.
7. Next, rotate your head to the left side.
8. Repeat the movement in the opposite direction.

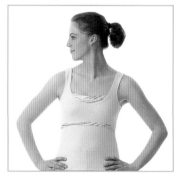

SHOULDER ROTATION

Benefits: This exercise helps to open up and tone tight shoulder and upper back muscles.

Note: You don't need to try to make the circles too big. The joints shouldn't click or feel strained, and your shoulders shouldn't hunch. Imagine you are oiling the insides of the shoulder joints.

1. Put both hands on the shoulders and stretch the elbows forward.
2. Inhale and lift the elbows to your shoulder's height.
3. Make a large circular motion and rotate them slowly one time. Exhale as you bring the elbows down.
4. Repeat six times front to back and six times back to front.

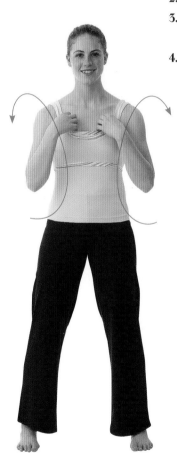

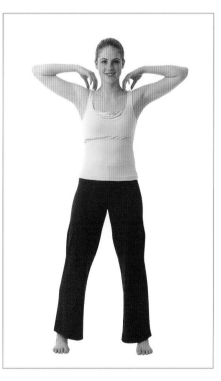

STANDING STRETCH

Benefits: This exercise stimulates the energy channels on the back side of the body and enhances blood circulation to the heart. It stretches the arm and shoulder muscles, and optimizes the function of the liver and other organs.

Note: Breathe deeply in each position, and let yourself stretch a little further with each inhalation.

1. Put your feet together and clasp your hands together.
2. Breathing in, lift your hands with palms facing the sky until your arms are touching your ears on either side. Turn your palms toward the sky.
3. At the same time, lift your heels and tilt your head backward to look at your hands.
4. Lower your hands slowly as you breathe out.
5. Repeat the motion with your arms raised and palms up. Inhale and tilt your whole body to the right side as far as it can go without losing your balance. Hold your breath and feel your whole left side being stretched.
6. Lower your hands and return to the upright position as you breathe out.
7. Repeat the motion, now moving to the left. Feel your whole right side being stretched.
8. Lower your hands and return to the upright position as you breathe out.
9. Breathe in as you bend forward at your waist and try to touch the ground with your palms. Be careful not to bend your knees. Try to touch your knees with your forehead, or come as close as you can.
10. Return to the starting position as you breathe out.
11. Repeat the whole cycle four times.

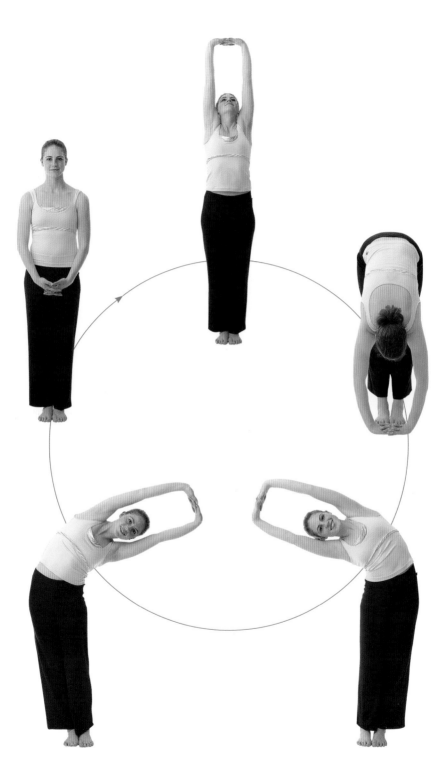

HIP ROTATION

Benefits: This exercise helps strengthen the hips and works the buttocks and hamstrings.

Note: As you do these exercises, it is most important to feel the area surrounding the hip joint. Focus on each particular point when rotating your hip joints. Bring your mind to the inside of your legs, then the outside, and continue rotating in this fashion.

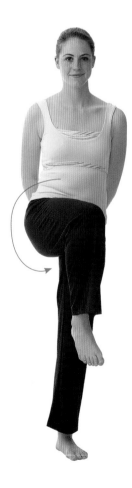

1. Relax the upper body and gently curl up the tailbone while standing up straight. When doing this motion, create firm but gentle tension in the lower abdomen.
2. In an "at ease" posture, lift the right knee up to the lower Dahn-jon level and rotate outward 10 times.
3. Change legs and do the same motion 10 times.
4. Lift the right knee again and rotate it 10 times in the opposite direction. Change legs and do the same motion 10 times.
5. Relax the chest and rotate the hip joint while trying to make sure the feet do not touch the ground.

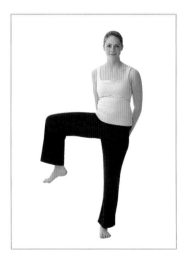

PELVIC ROTATION

Benefits: This exercise will train the muscles in your waist, buttocks, hips, thighs, and legs.

Note: Relax the chest and rotate the pelvis while keeping the upper body straight.

1. Stand with your feet apart and knees slightly bent, making sure that your hips don't slip backwards.
2. Spread the legs as wide as possible and assume the horse stance so that the ligaments in the hip joint can be stretched.
3. Rotate the pelvis and hip 10 times from left to right. Concentrate on the sensation of the pelvic movement and on exhalation.
   Keep the knees and chest stationary.
4. Reverse, rotating 10 times from right to left.

KNEE ROTATION

MERIDIAN STRETCHING

Benefits: This exercise promotes optimal blood and energy circulation in the knee joints. It also helps to relieve pain in the knee.

Note: While you are rotating the knees, do not let the bottom of your feet lift off the ground. Do not put any weight on your knees with your hands. Relax your upper body fully and have your weight rest only below the knees.

1. Place the knees together and massage your knees and knee caps with your hands.
2. Slightly bend your knees and keep the bottom of your feet flat on the floor. Do not put any weight on your knees with your hands. Relax your upper body.
3. Keep your knees together as you rotate your knees in a circular motion toward the right. Do not let the bottom of your feet lift off the ground.
4. Repeat the same movement in the opposite direction.
5. Rotate your knees inside to outside.
6. Repeat the movement in the opposite direction.

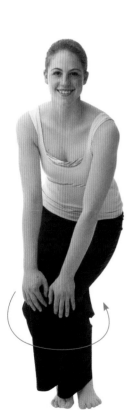

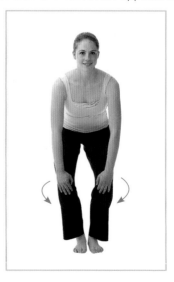

SIDE STRETCH

Benefits: This gives an excellent stretch to the spine, toning the spinal nerves and promoting proper function of the digestive system. This exercise also stretches out the part of the Liver Meridian that runs along the inner thighs to release blockages and to enable smooth energy flow.

Note: Take several full breaths in each position before releasing it for further stretching and relaxation.

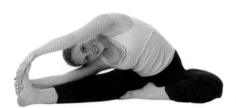

1. Sit up and stretch your right leg out to the side. Bend your left leg and tuck it in.
2. Place your right hand behind the arch of your right foot. Breathe in and stretch your left arm up and bend from the waist as you reach your hand over to your right foot. Hold for as long as comfortable while focusing on stretching your left side as much as possible. Exhale and return.
3. Repeat on the opposite side. Repeat each side at least twice.

4. Sit up with your spine straight and spread your legs.
5. Place your right hand on the left side of your rib cage. Breathe in and bend from the waist as you bring your hand over to your right foot. Hold for as long as is comfortable while focusing on stretching your left side as much as possible. Exhale and return.
6. Repeat on opposite side. Repeat each side at least twice.

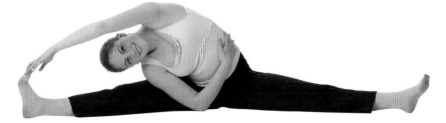

SITTING FORWARD BEND

Benefits: This exercise opens the energy channels on the back side of the body and stretches the whole body from the heels to the top of the spine.

Note: Don't try to bring your head to your knees as this will curve your spine. Instead, aim to bring the torso as far forward as possible, while keeping the knees and spine straight.

1. Sit with your legs together, stretching them straight out in front of you.
2. Place your hands on your knees. Bring your arms in a circular motion toward the back of your hips, circling them up overhead.
3. Inhale and bend your torso so that your hands can touch your toes. Concentrate on keeping your legs straight. Bend at the elbow, bringing your chest and head toward your knees. Exhale and return to the original posture.
4. Repeat this several times.

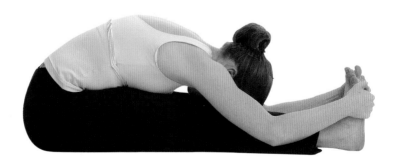

STRADDLE WITH FORWARD BEND

Benefits: This exercises stretches and lengthens the natural curve of the spine and hamstrings. It squeezes the abdominal organs and nourishes them with fresh blood and energy.

Note: Be sure to avoid overstretching your thighs by taking most of your weight on your hands at first. Little by little inch your way forward until you can bring your elbows down.

1. Stretch your legs apart as much as you can.
2. Point your toes upward.
3. Bend your elbows while leaning slightly forward with your palms down and your fingers facing each other. Bounce several times.
4. Bend more from your upper torso, trying to touch your chest and chin to your thighs while facing straight ahead. Touch your ankles with your hands.
5. Repeat several times.

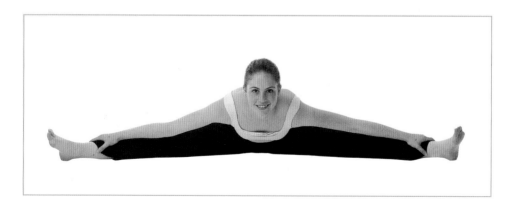

TOE TAPPING

Benefits: This exercise helps circulation to the lower extremities and balances water and fire energy in the body. It will also help provide a deeper and more peaceful sleep. Try this exercise just before bedtime if you suffer from insomnia.

Note: You can perform this exercise from either a lying or sitting position. You may place your hands on your abdomen or on the floor with palms facing upward.

1. Lie down on your back with your feet together.
2. Flex your feet and keep your heels together.
3. Tap your big toes together, then open your feet so that your little toes tap the floor. Repeat as rapidly as you can.
4. Begin with 100 repetitions and increase the number as you practice more.

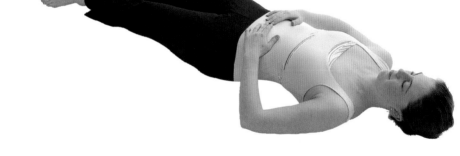

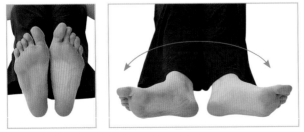

ROLLING BACK

Benefits: This exercise lengthens and strengthens the muscles of the spine. It enhances the nervous system and promotes optimal functioning of the vital organs in the body.

Note: Let your neck rhythmically follow the motion without pushing with your head. This is best performed on a lightly cushioned surface.

1. Sit with your knees bent and clasp your arms around your knees. Round your spine to form a C shape. Slightly lower your head. Relax your neck and your shoulders.
2. Gently roll back with your back softly touching the floor in order to stimulate your spine. Slowly and gently return to Step 1.
3. Repeat 10 times.

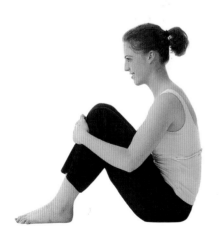
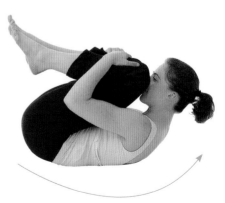

ABDOMINAL CLAPPING

Benefits: Abdominal Clapping is a simple but effective method for strengthening the lower abdomen, especially the Dahn-jon. By rhythmically patting the lower abdomen with the palms of both hands, blood and energy is distributed throughout the entire body. Abdominal exercises will assist in the prompt removal of excess gases and waste from the body, and you will feel increased warmth in the Dahn-jon, as well.

Note: Begin with 100 strikes. You may increase the number and force of the strikes with more practice.

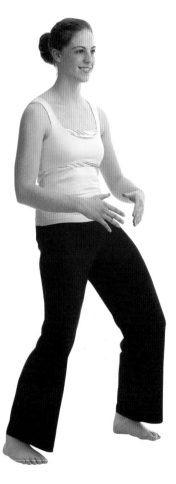

1. Spread your feet shoulder-width apart and bend your knees slightly.
2. Lengthen and relax your spine. Relax your shoulders, neck, and arms.
3. Point your toes slightly inward and feel a slight tightening of the lower abdomen.
4. Rhythmically strike the lower abdomen area with both palms.

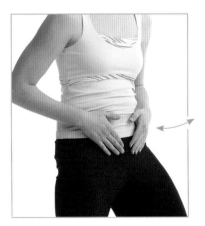

INTESTINE EXERCISE

Benefits: This exercise will increase the flexibility of the intestines and facilitate efficient circulation of both energy and blood. If you also tighten your rectal muscles during this exercise, you will be able to gather energy and feel warmth much more quickly.

Note: You should not overdo this exercise in the beginning since it may result in some discomfort.

1. This exercise can be performed standing up or lying down. When standing up, assume the same position as the abdominal clapping position (knees slightly bent, toes turned slightly inward). When lying down, lie on your back with your legs shoulder-width apart. Form a triangle by touching your thumbs and forefingers together and place them lightly on the lower abdomen.

2. When pulling in, pull as if the front wall of your abdomen is trying to touch your back. Tighten your rectal muscles at the same time.

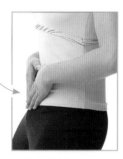

3. Then, push your lower abdomen out slightly, making it more round. You will feel outward pressure in your lower abdomen.

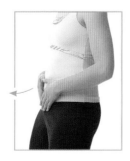

4. Repeat the movement. Start with one set of 50 and work your way up to a set of 300 as you advance.

WHOLE BODY STRETCH

Benefits: This exercise strengthens the abdominal muscles, stretches the spine and back muscles, and enriches blood circulation. The swinging movement keeps the intestines in their proper placement and shape and relieves constipation.

Note: This stretch is most often used as a finishing exercise because of its energizing effect. It's good to do just after Jung-Choong Breathing postures.

1. Lie on your back and lock your fingers together. Breathe in and extend both arms above the head. Point the toes downward and stretch the entire body. Exhale and relax. Repeat three times.
2. Now flex your toes and shift your arms and legs to the left side and then to the right side. Synchronize your movements so that your upper and lower body move together.
3. Keep your feet together as you perform these movements. Repeat several times.

MERIDIAN STRETCHING

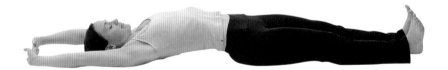

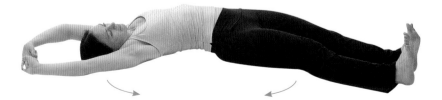

CROSSING LEGS TO FINGERS

Benefits: This exercise limbers the legs and hips, relieves tension in the back and torso, and increases spinal flexibility. It also tones abdominal muscles and massages a number of internal organs, including the liver and intestines.

Note: Do not twist your lower back or pelvis further than is comfortable. Stop if the pose causes any pain.

1. Lie on your back with arms extended to the side. Inhale. Lift your left leg to form a 90-degree angle.

2. Continue to hold your breath while crossing your left leg to touch your right fingers. Simultaneously, shift your eyes to the left and gaze at your left hand.

3. Exhale. Return to Step 1. Perform on the opposite side. Repeat twice.

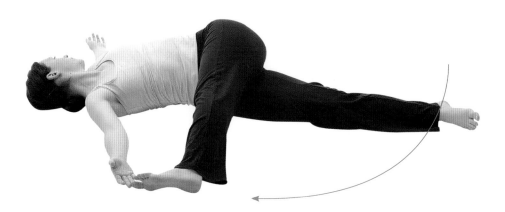

LIFTING LEGS OVER HEAD

Benefits: This exercise stretches the whole body and strengthens the back, shoulder, and arm muscles while releasing tension. It also increases the flexibility of the spine in both the back and neck and massages the internal organs by compressing the abdomen.

Note: When you practice this stretch, make sure to keep your spine pushed up and your knees straight.

1. Lie comfortably on your back.
2. Place your hands on the floor with palms face down, as shown in the picture. Inhale. Keep your feet together and slowly raise them off the floor, lifting your legs over your head with your toes touching the floor behind your head.
3. Hold this position for a few seconds. Exhale and return to Step 1. Repeat three times.
4. You can maintain this posture by supporting your lower back with your hands or holding your feet with your hands.

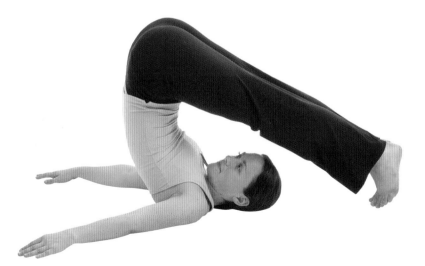

UPPER BODY LIFT

Benefits: This exercise strengthens the lower back and the lower torso with a powerful backward stretch as the abdominal organs are toned up and massaged. This works well as a finishing exercise.

Note: Follow this exercise very carefully and gently if you suffer from lower back pain.

1. Lie on your stomach, as shown in the picture. Place your arms on either side of your shoulders, with your palms touching the floor. Inhale and slowly raise your upper body.
2. As you raise your upper body, raise your head up and hold it in this position while concentrating on your spine.
3. Exhale and return to Step 1. Repeat several times.

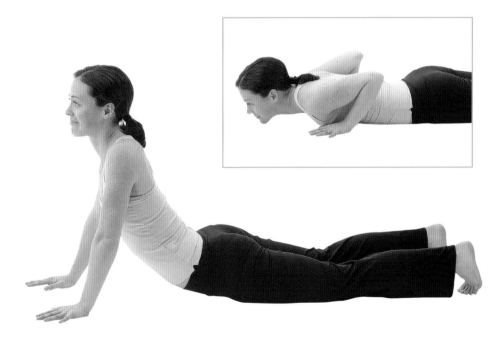

Having cast my body into the Void on the flow of Ki, I fill the Void to the brim. With Ki circulating throughout my body, the Cosmic Mind enjoys me and I enjoy the mind of the cosmos. My heart overflows with harmony and I have an earnest desire to circulate that Mind throughout the world.

—Ilchi Lee

Jung-Choong Breathing

Jung is a Korean word meaning vital energy, while *Choong* refers to fulfillment. Ideally, the process of breathing creates life energy, which is then accumulated in the Dahn-jon. However, this doesn't happen all the time. Why? Because the body is not properly positioned to gather the energy.

To gather energy, the outflow valve of the energy has to be closed. The hip joint, in conjunction with the tailbone, works as the valve for energy flow in the human body. Curling up the tailbone is very important because it helps to form a proper angle for gathering energy while causing a light tension in the Dahn-jon. Once the appropriate body position is taken, Ki generated by breathing is naturally gathered at the Dahn-jon. This gathered energy creates natural pressure around the abdomen, allowing proper energy circulation to happen naturally.

Another important benefit of Jung-Choong Breathing postures involves a core energy principle called "Water Up, Fire Down." As the Dok-maek, or Governing Meridian, that runs along the back is opened through the postures, cool water energy from the kidneys flows up easily to the head. In turn, by opening the Im–maek, or Conception Meridian that runs down the front of the body, hot fire energy from the chest is carried down toward the abdomen. As a result, the healthy energy state known as "Water Up, Fire Down" is restored.

Focus on Natural Breathing

For deep and natural breathing, the blockage around the chest caused by stress has to be opened. Breathe naturally, focusing on the exhalation. Relaxing your chest and upper body will help you. To open up the blockages, exhale with the mouth open slightly at the beginning stage, making a "ha-ah" sound through the throat to deeply release stagnant energy from the inside of the chest. After a certain time of exhaling this way, you may breathe with the mouth closed. As for the principles, Jung-Choong Breathing is not very different from the traditional breathing techniques. The distinction of Jung-Choong Breathing lies in its focus on natural breathing in a proper position instead of concentration on and intentional control of breathing.

The Importance of the Tailbone

Your tailbone is one of the most overlooked parts of the body, yet its position during your training exercises is the key to achieving optimal physical and mental well-being.

Jung-Choong Breathing embodies postures and breath work. It focuses on exhalation and proper positioning, letting inhalation happen naturally, without any conscious, intentional control. The angle of the tailbone is critical to the flow of energy in the body. Just as the internal organs are supported by the tailbone, so is our energy system.

In the embryonic stage, we all have a tail, but it is soon enveloped by the body as it enters the fetal stage of development. So, in fact, you still have a tail now, but it is inside your body, in the form of your very important but largely misunderstood tailbone.

You may have learned in biology that the human tailbone is "vestigial," meaning that it is an evolutionary "leftover," with no practical use for the modern human body. As it turns out, the tailbone is very important for the structure and support of the body—and the flow of energy throughout it.

First of all, the human tailbone acts as a cushion for the spine. The tailbone is actually constructed of three to five bones that are loosely hinged together. Whenever we sit down, the three bones curl under, acting as a shock absorber to protect the spine.

The tailbone also supports internal organs because many of the muscles that support the abdomen connect to it. Essentially, the muscles of the

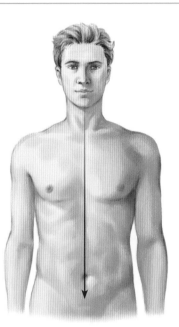

Im-maek

Hot fire energy flows down toward the abdomen through the Im-maek.

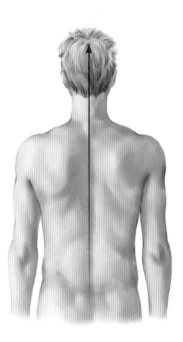

Dok-maek

Cool water energy flows up to the head through the Dok-maek.

lower abdominal cavity form a "hammock" that supports all the surrounding organs, attaching on the front to the forward pelvis and on the back to the lower spine and tailbone.

In the past, our ancestors placed great importance on the tailbone and its accompanying structure, the sacrum. The sacrum is the larger, flat bone above the tailbone that attaches the spine and tailbone to the pelvis, thereby forming the structural base of the body.

The word sacrum is Latin for "holy," and it was often referred to as the "holy bone." This originates from the notion that the sacrum forms the foundation of the human body and is therefore sacred on some level. Interestingly enough, the sacrum and tailbone are the last components of the body to degrade after death.

The lower Dahn-jon is the physical energy center located in the center of the lower abdomen, just in front of the sacrum. Regular Dahn classes focus on the development of this energy center. The middle and upper Dahn-jons are also important, but the lower center must be developed first in order to create a strong energetic center for the individual.

Curling the tailbone creates a bowl in which energy in the Dahn-jon can accumulate. By tilting the tailbone inward and upward at a concave angle, or curving it like the inside of a bowl, the energy of the lower Dahn-jon is contained.

Tensions in the body begin in the muscles around the base of the spine and then affect the rest of the body. By curling the muscles around the tailbone at a proper angle to gather energy while maintaining slight tension to the Dahn-jon, the spine straightens and sends energy all the way up to the brain, thereby revitalizing the entire body.

The key lies in tilting the tailbone at just the right angle. Curling up the tailbone is also very important because it helps to form a proper angle for gathering energy while causing a light tension in the Dahn-jon. As energy rises from the tailbone to the head, it activates the body's natural self-healing process. The important thing to remember when practicing this posture is to relax the entire body, especially the shoulders and legs. Tensing them will only close the "valve" and shut down the flow of energy.

When the hip joint is working in conjunction with the tailbone, it serves as the valve for the energy flow in the body. The hip joints should not be

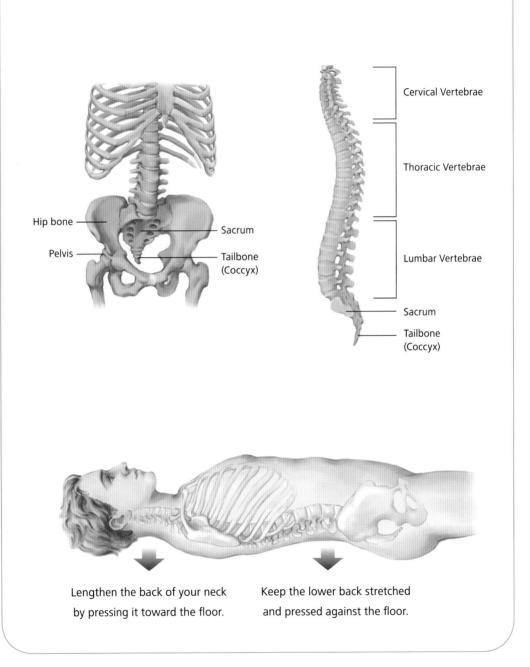

Hip bone
Pelvis
Sacrum
Tailbone (Coccyx)

Cervical Vertebrae
Thoracic Vertebrae
Lumbar Vertebrae
Sacrum
Tailbone (Coccyx)

Lengthen the back of your neck by pressing it toward the floor.

Keep the lower back stretched and pressed against the floor.

left open by letting the knees and thighs fall to the side. If your legs remain too far apart, the "valve" is open and the energy will flow out. To gather it, the outflow valve must be closed by maintaining the proper angle of the hip joints. This process helps to enhance the body's stability and to coordinate its functions.

Jung-Choong Breathing and Dahn-jon Breathing

Deep breathing occurs naturally if we breathe with our awareness focused on our Dahn-jon. As you do your breath-work, focus your mind on this area of your body. Feel your lower abdomen rising when you breathe in and falling when you breathe out. Do this slowly and concentrate on your breathing. This approach is called Dahn-jon breathing or abdominal breathing.

Dahn-jon breathing is closely related to the movement of the diaphragm, a dome-shaped structure that assists in breathing and acts as a natural partition between your heart and lungs on the one hand, and your stomach, spleen, pancreas, liver, kidneys, bladder, and small and large intestines on the other.

When you breathe deeply, your diaphragm moves downward as you inhale and upward as you exhale. The more the diaphragm moves, the more our lungs are able to expand, which means that more oxygen can be taken in and more carbon dioxide can be released with each breath.

The diaphragm is attached to the lower rib cage and has strands extending to the lumbar vertebrae. When you breathe fully and deeply, the belly, lower rib cage, and lower back expand on inhalation, thus pushing the diaphragm down deeper into the abdomen. The same structures retract on exhalation. In deep Dahn-jon breathing, these rhythmic movements help to detoxify the inner organs, promote blood circulation, and pump fluid more efficiently through the lymphatic system.

When you do Dahn-jon breathing, at first there may not be any sensation in the Dahn-jon. This may be due to the energy channel being blocked or the sense of Ki not being fully developed. With practice, the warmth of the energy moving inside the abdomen will become apparent. When there is a feeling of the heat in the abdomen, the Dahn-jon has been identified. Concentrate on that point. As the awareness of the Dahn-jon increases, more energy and heat will be felt. The sense of heat may change into a magnetic or electric sensation.

When the Dahn-jon feels warm, imagine an energy ball in the Dahn-jon. Deepen the breathing and the energy ball will become larger. Soon the abdominal area will be filled with the ball of energy. Through Jung-Choong Breathing postures and techniques, our breathing can become natural, deep Dahn-jon breathing.

Chest Breathing

If your chest feels tight, try chest breathing before you start Jung-Choong Breathing. Lie comfortably on the floor face up, spread your legs to about the width of your shoulders, and move your arms to the sides, about 45 degrees from your body. Close your eyes and take three or four slow, even breaths while counting to four. Breathing out slowly through your mouth, exhale the energy, releasing the stuffy, restless feeling in your chest. Breathe out slowly, to a count of six. Exhale quietly, with your lips parted slightly. Once you become comfortable with this step, concentrate your awareness on the tips of your fingers as you exhale, imagining that energy congested in your chest goes out through the ends of your fingers. If lying down, picture the energy leaving your body through the tips of your toes, as well as fingers.

Jung-Choong Breathing Sequence

The Jung-Choong Breathing postures are most effective when you adjust the sequence of the postures to your own condition. For beginners, we recommend a 20-minute routine in which the practitioner decides on the duration of each posture. Switch between Postures No. 2, 3, and 4 for 15 minutes, according to your comfort level. A rough guideline is provided for beginners who are not sensitized to energy flow. The ideal sequence should be Posture 2→3→4→3→2, but do what feels most beneficial for your body. If you feel a sharp pain or it becomes too difficult to keep the posture, move on to the next one.

Energy, Meet Physiology

The autonomic nervous system governs most of our bodily functions and encompasses the sympathetic and parasympathetic networks.

The sympathetic nervous system activates the "fight or flight" response, triggering increased heart rate and blood pressure, sweating, inhibition of digestion, and release of energy stores for use by the large muscle groups. In contrast, the parasympathetic nervous system activates the functions of "rest and digest."

The vagus nerve is part of the parasympathetic nervous system, extending from the medulla in the brain to the base of the spine, forming a network of vital links to the heart, liver, lungs, and other major organs.

Most noteworthy about this vital nerve is the correlation between its function and the phenomena people experience when they activate the Water Up, Fire Down energy principle. There is reason to believe that many of the phenomena associated with principle, including warmth in the abdomen, calming of the heart, teary eyes, and watering mouth, represent increased parasympathetic activity—a rest-and-digest workout for our autonomic nervous system.

Other parasympathetic nerves control tear and saliva production, as well as the emptying of the bladder and rectum. To those who have experienced a Dahn Yoga class, these effects will sound similar to what happens when they bring their 'energy down' to the Dahn-jon.

Since the nerve roots of the parasympathetic system are limited to the base of the brain and the sacrum, one can speculate about a possible connection between muscular contractions in the tailbone area—a key technique in the postures for the Jung-Choong Breathing—and overall activity in the parasympathetic nervous system.

Studies show that many natural health practices, including deep abdominal breathing and acupuncture, can stimulate activity in the parasympathetic nervous system. So, the next time you feel energy flowing, remember that you might be helping to improve tone in your autonomic nervous system, too. Although further scientific research is needed, such synergistic exploration of energy principle and physiology can forge an expanded understanding of our bodies and minds.

[eyes]

Energy flow As water energy reaches the head, the brain is cooled and refreshed; stagnant energy and toxins are released through the mouth (yawns) and eyes (tears).

Parasympathetic activation Stimulation of lacrimal glands releases tears.

[heart]

Energy flow Heat in the heart is cooled as fire energy travels downward toward the abdomen. The mind returns to a stable state.

Parasympathetic activation Slows the heart rate.

[lungs]

Energy flow Breathing becomes deeper and calmer with less need of oxygen in the body. Proper breathing, especially with a focus on exhalation, enhances a smooth cycle of descending heat and rising coolness.

Parasympathetic activation Constricts airways in the lungs.

[liver]

Energy flow Energy begins to accumulate.

Parasympathetic activation Stimulates the liver for glucose uptake, allowing accumulation of energy stores.

——————— Parasympathetic Nerves

[mouth]

Energy flow Circulation of water energy in the head alleviates dry mouth.

Parasympathetic activation Stimulation of mouth glands produces saliva.

[stomach, pancreas]

Energy flow Fire energy travels down to facilitate abdominal organs.

Parasympathetic activation Stomach and pancreas release acids and enzymes that stimulate digestion.

[kidneys]

Energy flow Kidneys generate water energy from the fire energy that has gathered in the Dahn-jon.

Parasympathetic activation Increases blood flow to the kidneys.

[intestines]

Energy flow Fire energy settles in the lower abdomen and finds its "home" in the Dahn-jon.

Parasympathetic activation Stimulates contraction of intestinal smooth muscle, promoting absorption of nutrients and flow of bowel contents.

posture 1: **RELAXATION**

Purpose: Deeply relaxes the mind and body and releases tension in preparation for subsequent postures.

Concentration: Curl your tailbone gently upward and feel a gentle pressure in the lower abdomen.

Breathing: Relax the mouth and keep it gently open as you focus on exhalation. Let inhalation happen naturally without being conscious of it. Do not attempt to control your breath or the movement of the abdomen. Center on the sensation of emptying your body.

Time: Hold the posture three to five minutes, until your body relaxes and your breath deepens.

1. Lie down on your back on a hard and warm surface.
2. Squeeze your legs tightly together and then completely relax them. They will part naturally, about the width of one foot. The angle of your feet should be about 30 to 45 degrees from the floor.
3. Place your middle fingers very lightly on your Dahn-jon (two inches below your navel). Do not press down since the Dahn-jon is sensitive to the slightest sensation. Keep the elbows resting comfortably on the floor. If your elbows lift off the floor, allow the hands to slide down the sides of the abdomen until the elbows rest on the floor.
4. Relax your body completely, especially the upper body, chest, and shoulders.
5. Curl the tailbone gently up, letting the lower back touch the floor as much as possible. As your tailbone tucks in, imagine creating a bowl for your Dahn-jon to collect energy, trying your best not to tense your legs in order to do so. You will automatically feel slight tension in your lower abdomen.
6. Close your eyes and focus on the energy flow inside your body.

Mouth is relaxed and chin is slightly tucked in.

Middle fingers rest lightly on the Dahn-jon.

Eyes are closed.

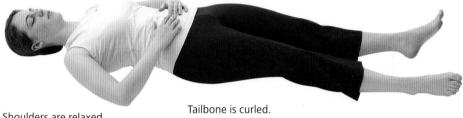

Shoulders are relaxed.

Tailbone is curled.

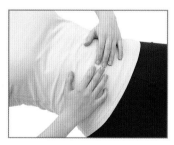

HAND POSITION

SELF CHECK •••••

1. Are your upper body and abdominal muscles relaxed?
➠ Relax the shoulders, chest, and solar plexus and straighten your spine.
2. Do you feel your lower back touch the floor?
➠ Try to find a sense of touching the floor with your lower back. Find a proper angle of your body that helps you breathe most naturally and comfortably.
3. Do you feel a slight tension in your abdomen or a sense of abdominal breathing?
➠ Move your energy in the upper body down to the abdominal area. With time and repeated practice, your breathing naturally progresses to a deep abdominal breathing.

posture 2: **ACCUMULATION**

Purpose: Accumulates energy in the Dahn-jon.

Concentration: Keep your tailbone curled, causing the whole back to touch the floor. As your Dahn-jon becomes filled with energy, this will gradually become easier.

Tip: To curl the tailbone in this posture, start by bringing your knees closer to your chest. Feel the tailbone lifting and the back touching the floor before readjusting the hips to a 90-degree angle.

Breathing: Close your mouth and start exhaling through your nose if it feels more natural. If that is uncomfortable, continue to exhale through your mouth.

Time: Three to five minutes. If holding the posture causes pain or becomes too difficult, change to the next posture.

1. Curl the tailbone upward, creating mild tension around the lower abdomen. Raise both legs with hips, knees, and ankles bent at a 90-degree angle.
2. Both the knees and ankles should be about one fist-width apart. Do not make the distance between the knees bigger than the distance between the ankles.
3. Keep both feet parallel. This helps to keep the hip joints in the correct position.
4. Flex your feet by pushing your heels out. Do not curl the toes as this creates blockages in the ankles.

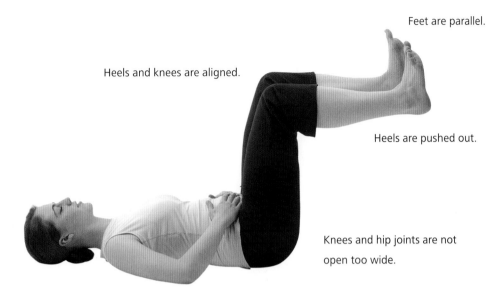

Feet are parallel.

Heels and knees are aligned.

Heels are pushed out.

Knees and hip joints are not open too wide.

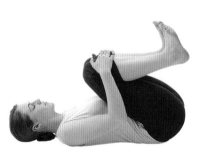

MODIFIED POSTURE

If holding this posture is difficult, pull your knees in toward your chest.

SELF CHECK •••••

1. Do you breathe slowly and comfortably?
➠ At first you may find that even holding the posture is difficult. However, with time and practice, you will breathe deeply and comfortably while holding the proper posture.
2. Can you feel your soles (Yong-chun) breathing?
➠ You may feel a stream of energy flowing out from your sole. It means that energy channels and points in your soles are activated.
3. How long can you hold this posture?
➠ Try to keep this posture more than 5 minutes without straining yourself.

posture 3: **CIRCULATION 1**

Purpose: Stimulates and opens the Bladder and Kidney Meridians, which run along the legs.

Concentration: Straighten the knees as much as possible.

Breathing: If breathing through the nose becomes easier than breathing with an open mouth, start breathing with mouth closed.

Time: Three to five minutes. If holding the posture causes pain or becomes too difficult, change to the next posture.

1. Firmly hold the front or sides of your feet. Slowly stretch and straighten both legs to the best of your ability.
2. Keep your head on the floor and your lower back as close to the floor as possible. The pelvis will lift off the floor. Vibration is likely to occur as the Bladder Meridian opens.
3. Completely relax your chest and shoulders.
4. Be sure to push out your heels to fully stretch the Bladder and Kidney Meridians.
5. If there is too much tension in the shoulders when you try to grab your feet, try the modified position (holding ankles or calves) to avoid tension in the shoulders.

Heels are pushed out to fully stimulate the meridians along the legs.

Keep knees straight (hold calves if necessary).

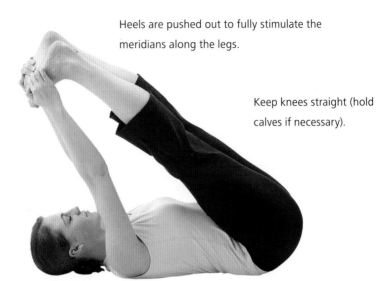

Shoulders are relaxed and as close to the floor as possible.

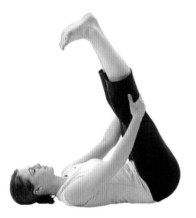

MODIFIED POSTURE

If you cannot straighten your legs completely while holding your feet, try holding the ankles, calves, or thighs, keeping your legs as straight as possible.

SELF CHECK •••••

1. Are you taking a proper posture and do you feel comfortable?
➠ Make sure your ankles are flexed enough and the backs of your legs are stretched.
2. Is your upper body relaxed?
➠ Relax your neck, shoulders, and chest area.
3. Do you feel that energy circulation is flowing through the Bladder Meridian?
➠ Starting at the eyes, the Bladder Meridian travels up over the crown of the head, and then flows down from the head along the back of the body to the toes. When you take a correct posture, the Bladder Meridian is activated, and you feel the energy flow along the pathway.

posture 4: **CIRCULATION 2**

Purpose: Opens the Im-maek and Dok-maek meridians that run along the front and back of the torso.

Concentration: Feel the stretch along the spine, even if this means you cannot keep your knees straight.

Breathing: Exhale slowly and comfortably while focusing on the spine.

Time: Three to five minutes. If holding the posture causes pain or becomes too difficult, change to the next posture.

Contraindications: Weak physical condition, pregnancy, obesity, or spinal disk injury. Avoid this posture and return to Postures 3 or 2.

JUNG-CHOONG BREATHING

1. From the previous posture, bring both legs completely over the head.
2. Keep the heels pushed out as you stretch and straighten the knees. If unable to straighten the knees, just flex your ankles back. It is okay if your toes float above the floor.
3. The arms should remain stretched out above the head, holding the feet in order to promote proper energy circulation.
4. Relax the shoulders as much as possible.
5. Focus on exhalation, not on the tailbone.

Keep knees stretched.

Ankles are flexed and heels are pushed out.

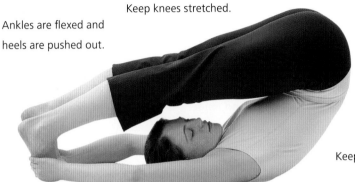

Keep your spine stretched.

Arms are stretched out above head.

SELF CHECK •••••

1. Are you breathing comfortably?
➠ Never hold your breath. Breathe naturally and focus on exhalation.
2. Is it too hard to take the posture?
➠ If you can't take the posture, then take circulation posture #1 or #2, the accumulation posture.
3. Do you feel stiff in the posture?
➠ Relax into the posture, focusing your mind on your breath. In this posture, it's better to exhale through your mouth.

posture 5: **RELAXATION AND ACCUMULATION**

Purpose: Opens the hip joints for relaxation and smooth energy flow.
Concentration: Feel energy accumulating in the Dahn-jon.
Breathing: Breathe deeply down to the lower abdomen.
Time: Hold the posture no longer than three to five minutes. You will feel your lower back become more relaxed and comfortable and your legs become very light. Continue to focus on your lower abdomen and watch your breath.

1. Bring your feet down to the floor with knees bent. Let the sides of your knees rest against each other.
2. Place your middle fingers lightly on the Dahn-jon.
3. Curl your tailbone, pushing your lower back comfortably to the ground.
4. Release tension from the shoulders and chest.
5. Breathe deeply and naturally. Notice your breath going down to your lower abdomen.
6. Feel energy accumulating in your Dahn-jon.

Upper body is relaxed.

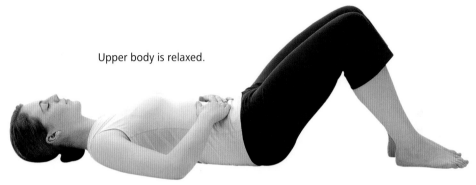

Release tension from the
chest and shoulders.

Keep your lower back as close to
the floor as possible.

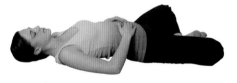

MODIFIED POSTURE

Fold legs in half or full lotus posture
and lower your legs to the floor. Or,
put the soles of the feet together and
relax your legs.

SELF CHECK •••••

1. Do you feel the tension in the upper body
   and the abdominal area?
   ➡ Relax, relax, and relax.
2. What kind of sensation do you feel in your
   abdomen?
   ➡ Breathe deeply and slowly from the
   abdomen, riding up and down on the
   breath, sinking deeper with each
   exhalation. Feel your abdomen expand
   and contract. You will feel warmth and a
   subtle feeling of energy in your Dahn-jon.
3. Is your breath deeper and softer than
   when you took the relaxation posture?

Everyday Jung-Choong Breathing

When we feel fatigued, we don't usually want to move our bodies, and we often decide to skip training. However, these times are when we need training most. When you feel you don't have enough strength to take the regular Jung-Choong Breathing sequence, try these modifications.

LEGS UP THE WALL ACCUMULATION

1. Lie on your back with your buttocks close to a wall and your legs elevated and resting against the wall.
2. Place your hands on your Dahn-jon.
3. If this pose causes discomfort due to tight hamstrings, move your buttocks a few more inches away from the wall.
4. Stretch and straighten both legs up to the best of your ability. Flex your feet and push out your heels.
5. Keep your head on the floor and your lower back as close to the floor as possible.
6. Close your eyes and focus on the energy flow inside your body.

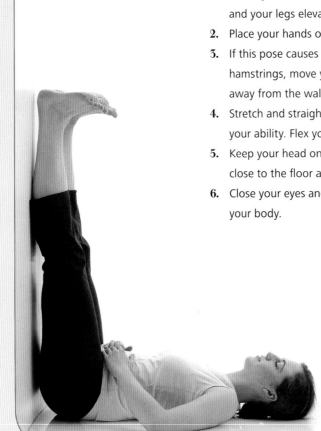

ACCUMULATION IN A CHAIR

1. Sit on a chair comfortably with your legs shoulder-width apart.
2. Place your hands on your Dahn-jon.
3. Relax your chest, shoulders, and arms completely.
4. You may close your eyes or leave them open.
5. Open your mouth slightly and keep focusing on exhalation. Focus on the energy flow inside your body.

CIRCULATION IN A CHAIR

1. Sit on a chair comfortably with your legs shoulder-width apart.
2. Bend your upper body from the waist and relax your upper body completely.
3. Rest your arms at your sides and be sure to relax them.
4. Open your mouth slightly and keep focusing on exhalation. Focus on the energy flow inside your body.

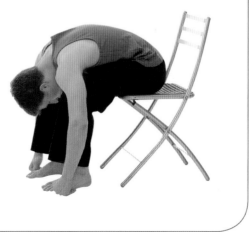

_____

We live with many thoughts, emotions, and habits, but at the same time we have other eyes, another mind capable of watching all these things. Those who practice self-cultivation find that mind; they live with it and they die with it.

　　　　　—Ilchi Lee

DahnMuDo

DahnMuDo is a comprehensive system of movement that is derived from the 5,000-year tradition of Korean healing and martial arts forms. DahnMuDo includes principles and practices for the enhancement of life energy and for the development of the ability to use energy. With the enhanced energy awareness gained through consistent training, practitioners can heal themselves physically and energetically.

Another phrase used to describe DahnMuDo is "the art of being limitless." The word *dahn* means "energy"; *mu* means "limitless"; and *do* means "the way." Thus, it is a discipline designed to develop power and to uncover endless creative energy. Through diligent practice, practitioners work to attain unlimited awareness, which is the true source of personal freedom and creativity.

Although DahnMuDo is a form of martial art, it is not used to compete or fight with an opponent. Rather, it is designed to enhance personal strength and integrity. The ultimate goal of DahnMuDo is to develop a complete human being who has full mastership of body, mind, and spirit.

While many DahnMuDo forms can be physically challenging, it is gentle enough to be practiced by anyone of any age. The speed, strength, intensity, and height of particular moves might be different for each individual practitioner, but the forms are intentionally designed to avoid injury to the body, unlike other combative martial art forms. It is said that the ideal age for practice is from eight to 88.

Dedicated students of DahnMuDo experience many forms of DahnMuDo training, including non-combative kicks, punches, and sword work. However, in regular Dahn Yoga training, we focus on the seven sets of Un-ki-bo-hyung-gong, a fundamental form of DahnMuDo. This is a method of training that adds hand movements to leg forms (Bo-hyung) to grow stability and strength in the lower body. Furthermore, the postures develop and stimulate the hemispheres of the brain, as left and right sides of the body move with balance and coordination.

These postures also promote proper circulation of energy throughout the body. The training for each set is generally done for about one minute by beginners and for about three to five minutes once practitioners are more comfortable with the postures. When moving from one set to the next, practitioners transition smoothly between postures, moving like water as they flow with universal energy. Since it trains the lower body so intensely, Un-ki-bo-hyung-gong also helps to build the Dahn-jon, the center of physical energy. This, in turn, leads to greater centeredness and clarity of mind.

Mastery

Pull back but do not shrink
Spread out but do not explode
Upper body as soft as the spread of mountains
Lower body as strong as a forest of sycamores
The power created by softness and strength
Movement and stillness
Inside and outside
Yin and yang
Flows deep into bones

The subtle harmony of bends and curves
Of the body reaching toward heaven
Of the body rooted in the earth

Unnoticed, the body disappears
The mind disappears
And even I, filled with energy, disappear

Only the clear, bright world remains
Reflected in the tranquility

—*Ilchi Lee*

Basics of DahnMuDo

The upper body must be kept very light and comfortable and centered at the navel. In the lower body, the hip joints must be relaxed and the body's weight must be distributed evenly so that it rests solidly over the soles of both feet. For lower body training, practitioners work to hold one posture for extended periods of time. Holding a posture for a long time causes respiration to deepen and energy to collect in the Dahn-jon. Before beginning the seven sets of Un-ki-bo-hyung-gong, a person lays the foundation for later training through Waist-Hip Rotation and Chuk-ki Stance (energy accumulation training).

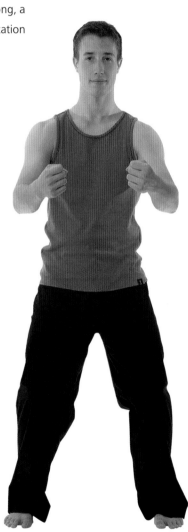

WAIST-HIP ROTATION

1. Stand with your feet parallel and shoulder-width apart.
2. Make relaxed fists with both hands and bring them to chest height.
3. Gently tuck in your tailbone as you bend your knees slightly.
4. Imagining that a weight is hanging from your tailbone, rotate only the area below your navel to the right in a circle. Do 20 repetitions.
5. Switch directions and do 20 more repetitions.

CHUK-KI STANCE

1. Stand with your feet shoulder-width apart and parallel. Make sure that your weight is distributed evenly so that it rests firmly over the soles of both feet.
2. Gently tuck in your tailbone.
3. Relaxing your upper body, raise your hands to chest height, and spread them apart about one foot.
4. Imagine that you have a ball of energy between your hands and your chest.
5. Concentrate on your Dahn-jon and maintain this posture for about 5 to 10 minutes.

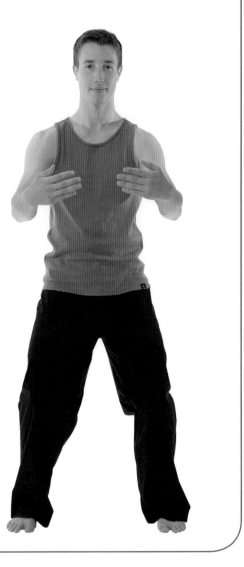

Bow Stance: **GUNG-JEON-BO**

Introduction: In Gung-jeon-bo, or Bow Stance, your front leg is curved like a bow and your back leg is straight like an arrow. The point of this stance is to feel the contractive pressure on the pelvis and to correctly align the angle of the hip joints. It straightens the lower back, adjusts the spine and pelvis, and develops the strength of the back part of the thigh, spreading energy to the whole body.

Set: The front leg should be held so that the shin is perpendicular to the ground and the back leg should be held with the knee extended straight and the heel touching the ground. The body is held erect and the lower back kept straight like an arrow notched in a taut bow string. The front leg supports the upper body and keeps it from leaning; the back leg presses firmly into the ground for support.

If the left foot is in front, this stance is called Jwa-gung-bo (Left Bow Stance); if the right foot is in front, it is called U-gung-bo (Right Bow Stance).

1. Move your hands in front of your chest and position them as if holding a ball.
2. Take one step forward with your left foot and use your hips to press down lightly on the sole of your foot.
3. Bend your left leg so that your shin is perpendicular to the floor and straighten your right leg, locking your knee and pressing downward into the floor with the heel of your foot.
4. With both hands positioned at the center of your body and your elbows slightly bent, extend your right hand and bring your left hand below your right elbow. Your hands and feet are positioned opposite to each other at this time.
5. Now, repeat the same motion on the other side.

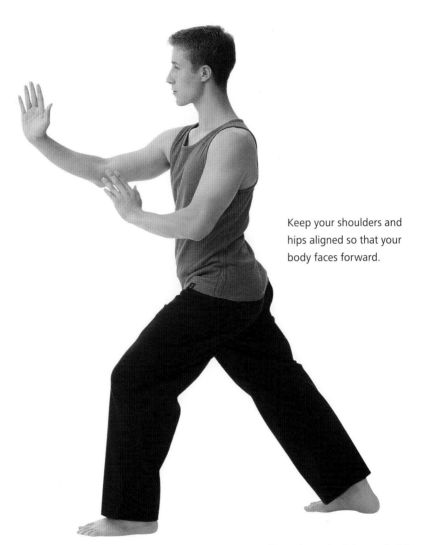

Keep your shoulders and
hips aligned so that your
body faces forward.

Place the big toe of your front foot and the
heel of your back foot on a straight line.

Extend your back leg so that its
strength passes your thigh and rises
to your shoulders and back.

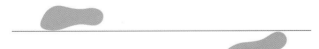

Horse Stance: **KI-MA-BO**

Introduction: Stand with your feet parallel and bend your knees so that your whole body's weight rests firmly over the soles of both feet. This stance is very effective for bringing energy down to the Dahn-jon as you concentrate your awareness there, taking advantage of the weight-bearing power of your feet.

Set: Spread your feet about one-and-a-half to two shoulder-widths apart and bend your knees. Ensure that your lower back is straight and that your upper body does not lean to the left or right. Align your feet so that they are parallel. Distribute your weight evenly over both feet and lower your center of gravity.

1. From the last movement of Gung-jeon-bo, position your hands in front of your chest as if holding a ball and turn your body 90 degrees to the left.
2. Spread your feet apart so that they are parallel to each other and bend your knees, adopting a Ki-ma Stance, as if riding a horse.
3. Lower your hands to your Dahn-jon.
4. Rotate your palms outward as you draw an oval with your hands, moving them from your Dahn-jon to chest height.
5. Spread your hands about one foot apart.

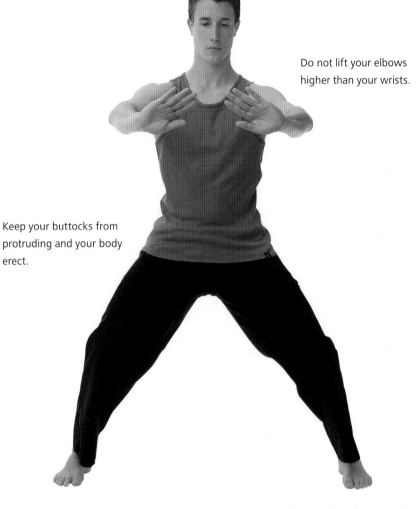

Do not lift your elbows higher than your wrists.

Keep your buttocks from protruding and your body erect.

Make sure that the outer edge of your foot does not lift off the ground.

Empty Stance: **HEO-BO**

Introduction: This set allows Ki energy to be accumulated very quickly. The balance of your stance should not be disturbed even if you lift your front foot off the ground. It rapidly strengthens the Dahn-jon in your lower abdomen and develops your body's quickness and resilience. However, this stance should not be held for long if it results in pain or excessive fatigue.

Set: Point the toes of your back foot about 30 degrees to the outside, bend your knee and sit into the stance with your weight over your back leg. Slightly bend your front leg, raising your front heel and lightly touching the big toe of your front foot to the ground. Place your weight only on your back leg. When the left foot is in front, this stance is called Jwa-heo-bo; when the right foot is in front, it is called U-heo-bo.

1. Shift your weight to your right leg.
2. Step forward with your left foot about 45 degrees.
3. At this time, place about 90 percent of your weight on your right leg and the rest on your left leg.
4. With both hands positioned at the center of your body and your elbows slightly bent, extend your left hand.
5. Bring your right hand below your left elbow.
6. Your hands and feet are positioned the same at this time (i.e., left hand and left foot forward, right hand and right foot back).
7. Position your hands as if you are holding a ball and return your feet to their original position.
8. Shift your weight to your left leg and perform the movement on the other side.

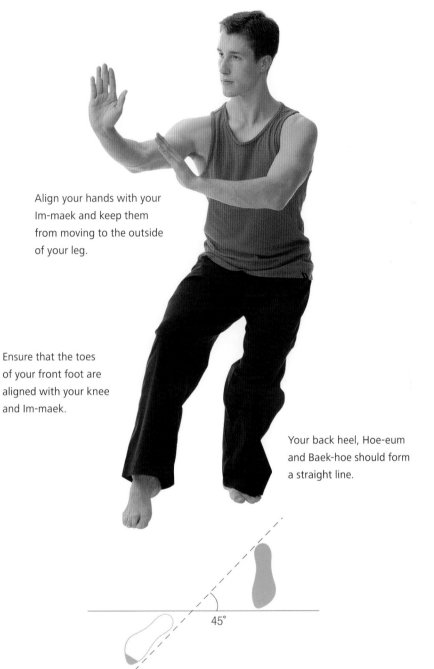

Align your hands with your Im-maek and keep them from moving to the outside of your leg.

Ensure that the toes of your front foot are aligned with your knee and Im-maek.

Your back heel, Hoe-eum and Baek-hoe should form a straight line.

45°

Single Leg Stance: **DONG-NIP-BO**

Introduction: Dong-nip-bo is a stance that has an air of aloofness, like a crane standing high, close to the sky. The stance is very good for meditation training and effective for improving concentration as well as mental stability. The body's weight remains balanced over one leg, with the foot gripping the floor. The other leg is held with the knee raised to form a right angle and the ankle relaxed.

Set: Stand on one leg and hold your other leg raised with knee bent. The leg you are lifting should be held so that your thigh is parallel to the ground. Extend your foot with your toes pointing toward the ground and positioned beside the knee of your supporting leg. The hand on the side of your raised leg should be held in a fist, with the arm rotated inward so that the fist points downward. The opposite hand should be held with the fist facing upward. When standing with the left foot in front, this stance is called Jwa-dong-nip-bo; when standing with the right foot in front, it is called U-dong-nip-bo.

1. From the last movement of Heo-bo, bring your right foot beside your left foot.
2. Bring your fists to your sides.
3. Extend your right arm, moving your right fist to the inside of your right thigh.
4. As you raise your right leg, extend your left fist skyward.
5. Look to the right and balance your weight over your left leg.
6. Slowly lower your hand and leg and then repeat the movement on the opposite side.

Bring the inside of your toe on the lifted leg back so that it touches the side of your other knee.

Ensure that your knee does not move to the outside.

Place your center of gravity over the big toe of the foot of the supporting leg.

Drop Stance: **BU-TOE-BO**

Introduction: Extending one leg stimulates the Gall Bladder Meridian, filling a person with confidence, and trains the hip joint; bending the other leg trains the thigh. Bu-toe-bo is a stance in which the distribution of strength in the legs must be maintained since they take very different shapes. It is effective for causing energy to sink in a stable way.

Set: Bu-toe-bo is adapted from Ki-ma-bo by bending one knee and sitting down on one leg while straightening the other leg. Make sure that the knee of the supporting leg does not come out of alignment with the toes of the foot below it. Your feet should be parallel, with the toes pointing the same direction. When the left leg is extended, the stance is called Jwa-bu-toe-bo; when the right leg is extended, it is called U-bu-toe-bo.

1. From the final movement of Dong-nip-bo, lower your left foot to your right ankle.
2. Dragging your left foot to the left, spread your feet shoulder-width apart.
3. Bend your right leg as if in a Ki-ma-bo and straighten your left leg.
4. Place your left fist just to the inside and lightly touching your right elbow. Move your right hand to make an oval shape.
5. Slowly spread your arms, with your right hand moving to the height of your right ear and your left hand moving downward at a 45 degree angle above your thigh.
6. On the opposite side, as you move your left hand into an oval shape, bend your left leg as if in a Ki-ma-bo and extend your right leg.

Look comfortably in the direction of your extended leg.

Bring the wrist of the hand you raised up to your shoulder on the same side.

Ensure that the lowered hand does not go beyond your thigh on the same side.

Apply strength equally to both legs, making sure that energy does not go more to one side than the other.

Keep your extended leg straight.

Sitting Stance: **IL-JWA-BO**

Introduction: In martial arts, this stance is used to advance forward while keeping the body low. It enhances agility because, after moving in, you may have to back out very quickly in a higher stance. Maintain the height of your knees so that they are not overstressed.

Set: Turn the tip of your front foot inward slightly and bend your knee so that your thigh is perpendicular to the ground. Bend your back leg and sit into the stance so that your back heel is raised, causing the bottom of your foot to form an angle of about 30 degrees from the ground. When the left leg is in back, this stance is called Jwa-il-jwa-bo; when the right foot is in back, it is called U-il-jwa-bo.

1. From Bu-toe-bo, pull in your left foot so that there is a distance of half a step between your feet.
2. Turn your body to the left so that you are facing the front.
3. Turn the big toe of your front foot inward about 5 degrees.
4. Brush your hands past your ribs, pressing forward. Tuck in your hips as you sit into the stance.
5. Lift your back heel so that the bottom of your foot forms a 45 degree angle from the ground.
6. Bring your hands back to your sides and perform the movement on the opposite side.

Extend palms forward,
wrists at shoulder height.

Keep your spine erect
so that your buttocks
do not protrude.

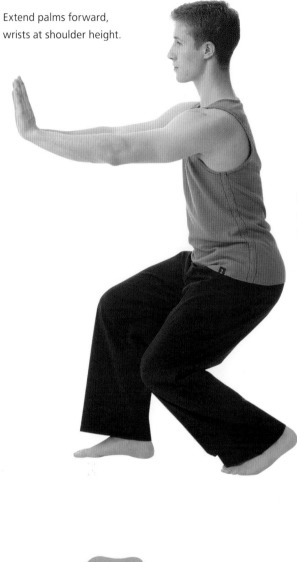

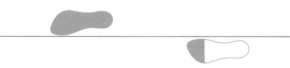

Cross Stance: **JWA-BAN-BO**

Introduction: This stance improves joint rotation. It strengthens the muscles in the legs and promotes active use of the lower back. It develops strength, agility, and flexibility. From Ki-ma-bo, turn as far as possible on the heel of one foot and the ball of the other foot and lower your stance.

Set: Cross your legs and turn the toes of the front foot outward as you bend your knee and sit into the stance. Bend the knee of your back leg, raising the heel of your back foot so that the bottom of the foot forms an angle of about 30 degrees from the ground. In this stance, the knee of the back leg is positioned close to the crook of the front knee. Keep your upper body erect and your lower back straight.

1. From the last position of Il-jwa-bo, bring your hands to your sides.
2. Turn your body to the left to create Ki-ma-bo.
3. From Ki-ma-bo, turn your left foot outward at least 180 degrees, pivoting on the heel.
4. Rotating your body, pivot on the ball of your back foot and bring your right knee into the crook of your left knee as you sit into the stance, with legs crossed.
5. Look to the front.
6. Open your fists and press downward with the base of your palms so that your arms form an angle of about 45 degrees from your body.
7. Bend and rotate your wrists inward so that your fingers turn toward your body.
8. Straighten your crossed legs as you return to face the front and then perform the movement on the opposite side.

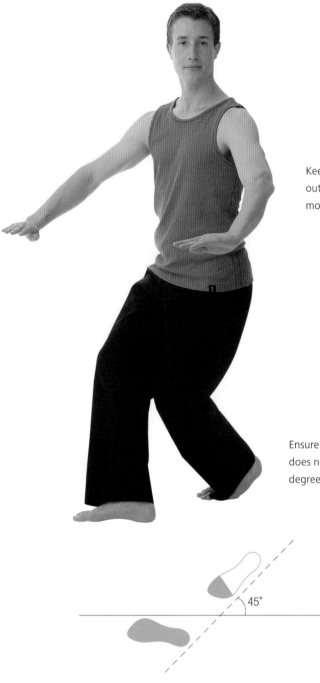

Keep the elbows of your outstretched arms from moving behind your back.

Ensure that your back heel does not lift more than 45 degrees off the ground.

45°

Sit down comfortably. As you control your breathing, have your mind watch your body. And tell yourself, "It's okay." Then your soul will find rest, and your body, too, will find comfort and new strength.

—Ilchi Lee

Meditation

When energy fills up the lower Dahn-jon, our bodies and minds are naturally revived. After practicing Jung-Choong Breathing and DahnMuDo, the circulation of energy and blood increases so that we can achieve a more deeply relaxed and meditative state.

Meditation involves focusing the mind and observing ourselves in the moment. It can take us deeper inside ourselves, beyond the illusions created by our thoughts and senses so that we can experience everything in its truest form. In short, meditation is nothing more than a stilling of the mind. Practitioners of Dahn Yoga are encouraged to do this through Ji-gam (energy sensitivity) training. The aim is to channel the mind's attention into a single focus, beginning with the feeling of energy between our hands. This sensation of energy later grows to include energy flowing through and around our whole body. Through careful concentration, we can subdue the endless stream of random thoughts the mind creates and become fully present in our body.

In Dahn Yoga, energy is used as a medium to focus on the breath. We sit in a half-lotus posture and slowly bring our hands up to face each other. Feeling the slight sensation between the hands requires all our concentration. When we cannot feel much, we are reminded that thoughts are energy, and that we have followed our thoughts instead of focusing between our hands. Do not follow the energy of your thoughts. Instead, center your attention between your hands. Build on the energy sensation between them, bringing them closer and then further apart, connecting your breathing to this movement.

Do not become frustrated with thoughts. The brain generates thoughts in the same way that the heart pumps blood. That is the function of the brain. You do not sit and worry about your heart doing what it is supposed to do. You wouldn't get angry with it for doing its job. Apply the same easy acceptance to the function of your brain. Let it send you thoughts. Just do not get carried away by them or show your interest in them.

If you lose your focus on the energy between your hands, there are two things you can do. If you find yourself distracted by a single stray thought, simply bring your mind back to the feeling between your hands. Do not take any more note of it; simply refocus. If you suddenly realize that the distraction has gone on for a while before you catch yourself, simply begin again. Allow distractions to come and go, without monitoring yourself. Eventually, mind, breath, and energy become one.

Once you are connected to your breath and energy, it is easy to return to your body. Most of the time, we experience life through our body without really being aware of that body. There is usually a web of busy inner dialogue running through our minds. We are usually so mesmerized by our ideas about the world that we miss out on much of the body's direct sensory experience.

In Dahn Yoga, we use the body as a tool to reawaken ourselves to sensations. Becoming aware of our physical sensations is a necessary prerequisite to mindfulness because such sensations are linked to feelings and thoughts, and they are the foundations of the very process of consciousness.

Being mindful of sensations in our body does not mean standing apart and observing like a distant witness. Rather, we directly experience what is happening in our bodies, and we carefully feel the energy that flows through them when we focus on them.

Awakening to our bodies allows us to experience the physical world fully, with all its anxieties, confusions, and pleasures, rather than living in a world of mere thoughts. Watching your body means asking yourself, "How does it actually feel to be anxious, angry, or happy? What is the texture of the experience?"

Meditation teaches us to stay with the bodily reality of the present moment, which offers us the possibility of seeing our life with a sense of clarity that we could never experience through thinking alone.

Chanting, breathing, or imagery is generally used in order to focus during meditation, along with Ji-gam training. The Ji-gam and Dahn-mu introduced below should be absorbed into meditation by concentrating on the energy sensation. Ji-gam and Dahn-mu are types of dynamic meditation that let the body move with the flow of energy. They especially help beginners concentrate more easily on the meditation. Vision meditation is for re-creating our lives by infusing our minds with positive thoughts, feelings, and imagery.

How to Still the Mind

Try the following methods, picking the one that suits you best and then practicing it consistently. Each of these methods produces its own unique, subtle feelings and energies. Whatever method you choose, it is important to deeply immerse yourself in the experience so you can feel its essence. Return to the object on which you were concentrating, without making any judgments about stray thoughts that creep into your mind. Even if thoughts continue to arise in the back of your mind, keep bringing the object on which you are focusing to the front of your mind.

CHANTING: This is a way to concentrate by repeating a special sound, phrase, or affirmation in your mind or out loud. It is very effective, especially for beginners, and relatively easy compared to other methods. Frequently, the Dahn Yoga phrase, "Chun-ji-ki-woon, Chun-ji-ma-eum (Cosmic Energy, Cosmic Mind)," is used for this purpose. Inwardly, repeat "Chun-ji-ki-woon" as you breathe in and "Chun-ji-ma-eum" as you breathe out. Repeating words that put your mind at ease and give you strength, such as "peace" and "love," or affirmations such as "I am relaxed" or "My body is not me, but mine" are also very effective.

BREATHING: To help you focus on breathing, try counting your breaths. Set a number in advance, such as 20 or 30 or 50, and count each breath. Once you reach that number, start over and begin counting again. Or say "one" as you slowly breathe in and "two" as you breathe out. When your mind is calmer, try to concentrate on the breathing itself. Carefully notice your breath coming in and going out, observing the nuances of your breathing and the changes taking place in your body. Notice the sound, length, and depth of your breathing, the movement of your abdomen and torso, as well as the temperature and energy you feel in your body. Beginners who have trouble concentrating can place one hand on their Dahn-jon and one hand on their chest. Notice the movement of the abdomen and torso, as well as the length, depth, and smoothness of the breath.

IMAGERY: This method involves visualizing a specific object or natural landscape. Commonly, we picture in front of our eyes the bright sun, a calm sea or lake, or a bouquet of flowers in full bloom, for example. Or we concentrate on one of the body's seven chakras (energy centers) and also visualize the color associated with that chakra. Practitioners usually concentrate on the lower Dahn-jon, which is equivalent to the second chakra located in the abdomen. Visualizing a red ball, the sun, or a candle will help to develop Dahn-jon awareness.

Meditation in Daily Life

Our meditation practice itself is the key to developing the mindfulness that lets us recognize the nuances of our lives. By becoming more aware of what we are actually doing during meditation – being more mindful of our bodies and minds—we can in turn be more aware in our everyday lives, even when we are not meditating.

When we become fully present, we experience moments of complete mindfulness. We set aside time for meals; we simplify our lives; we give our full attention to the task at hand. We do things with unbroken concentration. We mindfully choose what we read, watch, and listen to. We boldly act upon on our concern for a stranger's well-being without holding back. And we seek spiritual, inspirational wisdom at every opportunity.

By honing our skills in meditation, we become fully aware of the subtle changes that are a natural part of our lives. Embracing these changes allows us to be warm, funny, joyful, radiant, relaxed, and loving. Our improved attitude in turn affects our friends, family, and even strangers, and it leaves us in a place where healing begins—for ourselves and the world.

A comfortable and correct sitting posture speeds up your progress in meditation. Here, Ilchi Lee, founder of Dahn Yoga, introduces "The Art of Sitting":

Sit down with legs crossed in the half-lotus position. Close your eyes and straighten your lower back. Twist your body five or six times to the left and right. Find your body's center of gravity. Align the knees and tailbone to form a triangle. Think of your spine as a pillar erected on the base of this triangle. Your head sits atop this pillar. Imagine that your arms support this pillar at the left and right in order to keep your head in place. Completely relax your arms, feeling as if your hands are dangling from your trunk. Relax your neck and shoulders, and feel your head sitting very lightly atop your spine. Feel how light it is. It seems your head might fly away on a breeze.

Feel your eyes, ears, nose, and mouth attached to your head. Gently close your eyes. Your pupils will naturally point downward. Relax your eyelids. Feel the eyelids lightly covering your pupils, thin membranes like the wings of a dragonfly. Imagine there is another eye between your eyebrows. Imagine that this eye is open and looking at a light far off in the distance.

Normally, we are not aware of our sensory organs. We rarely think of our senses as separate from ourselves. This is why we are tricked into thinking that the phenomena we perceive through our senses are the substance of reality. Try to feel your "sensory self." Your "self," with eyes, nose, ears, thoughts, and emotions, is sitting here like this. Who is this "I" sitting here?

We feel greater dignity and confidence as our sitting posture becomes stronger and more developed. One side of your body is placed firmly on the ground and the other side is opened toward heaven. Feel your own holiness when you body links Heaven and Earth as one, like a tree with solid roots sinking into the ground and a majestic trunk stretching toward the sky.

Feeling Energy: **JI-GAM**

Relaxed concentration is an absolute prerequisite to being able to feel the flow of Ki energy. We usually tense up when we concentrate and let our thoughts wander without direction when we cease to concentrate. Therefore, relaxed concentration may sound like an oxymoron. However, only when we can direct our consciousness while maintaining a relaxed state of body and mind can we feel the flow of energy.

To feel the energy, we need to turn the focus of our consciousness inward. We must separate ourselves from our outer distractions, thoughts, and emotions. We call this process Ji-gam. The basic requirement for Ji-gam practice is determined concentration on the body here and now.

We begin Ji-gam training with our hands first because they are the most sensitive part of our body, allowing us to feel Ki energy most easily. When we are able to sense energy in our hands, it becomes easier to awaken this same sensitivity in other parts of the body, including the brain. Although the amount of time it takes to feel this energy for the first time varies from person to person, everyone will eventually succeed with enough practice.

When we become used to feeling energy in our hands, we can maintain the sensitivity and the feeling without having to be in a special position or environment. This also means that it is possible to function in the everyday world in a clearer and calmer state of consciousness.

1. Sit in a half-lotus position and straighten your back.

2. Place your hands on your knees with your palms facing up and close your eyes. Relax your body, especially your neck and shoulders. Relax your mind. Inhale deeply and let go of any remaining tension while exhaling.

3. Raise your hands slowly to chest level, with your palms facing each other but not touching. First concentrate on any sensation you may feel between your palms. You may feel warmth, tingling, or even your own pulse.

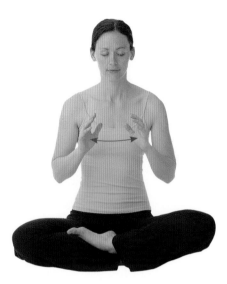

4. Now, part your hands about two to four inches and concentrate on the space between them. Imagine that your shoulders, arms, wrists, and hands are floating in a vacuum, weightless.

5. Pull your hands apart and push them closer in again as you maintain your concentration. Feel the energy flow between your palms.

6. When the sensation becomes more real, pull your hands farther apart and push them closer together. Feel the sensation expand and become stronger.

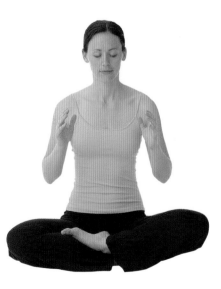

7. Breathe in and out, slowly and deeply, three times.

8. Rub your hands together briskly and gently sweep your face, neck, and chest.

Flowing with Energy: **DAHN-MU**

Dahn means "energy." *Mu* means "dance." Dahn-mu is a form of dancing with the natural flow of energy, called "the dance of Ki."

This gentle dancing is an effective method to control and utilize Ki. Practitioners usually experience Ki as a gentle vibration inside the body. The Ki usually begins in the hands and then quickly moves through the whole body until the entire body is responding in dance-like movements called Dahn-mu.

This exercise is particularly easy to accomplish since there is nothing to learn in the way of technique. The alignment of the body with Ki is influenced by the state of mind of the participant. The resulting Dahn-mu might be expressed with fast or slow motions and restrained or passionate movements. The expression of Ki may include complex and intricate movements that a person might not normally make. When the rhythmic flow of Ki is followed with movement, practitioners dance naturally, ignoring the long repressed and inhibited movements that they may have held in the past.

These graceful motions come from deep within a person's being as a perfect, spontaneous expression of vital energy. Out of these dance-like movements of self-expression, practitioners begin to experience a gentle, dynamic meditation from a subconscious state.

As the dancing progresses, practitioners will begin to feel joy and gratitude bubbling up from inside them. Tears may erupt, releasing blocked emotions locked in the chest. Experiencing Dahn-mu brings forth a true understanding of freedom. Allowing the spontaneous dance movements is the same as trusting the benevolent wisdom of energy. After realizing the way that Ki works, practitioners can easily gain control and utilize Ki at will.

1. Sit comfortably in a half lotus position.
2. Repeat the Ji-gam exercise and gradually increase the feeling of Ki.
3. While immersing yourself into the feeling of Ki through the motions of opening and closing the hands, you will feel the whole body move naturally. This is the beginning of Dahn-mu.
4. Let your body move naturally with the flow of the energy.
5. It is ideal to have background music that can naturally lead the body movement while practicing.

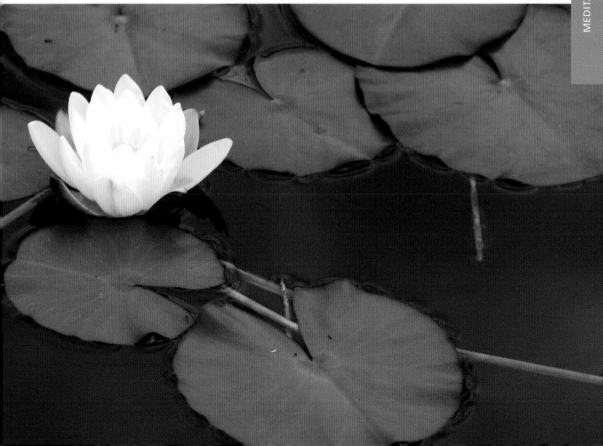

VISION MEDITATION

MEDITATION

Our brains sometimes can't distinguish between reality and imagination. Imagine that you're taking a bite of a very sour lemon right now. Although you actually didn't eat the lemon, you salivate. As you can see from this example, our thoughts and emotions directly impact our bodies. That is why it is important to focus your mind intently on what you would like to manifest in the world.

When you discover your desired goal, make up your mind firmly that you will make it so. Then imagine that you have already made it happen and believe that you will be there. Then keep making detailed action plans and challenge yourself endlessly until you can see the results.

During this process, belief in yourself and imagination play crucial roles. If you can vividly draw what you desire, then you can always find plenty of ideas to make it come true. The imagination plays such a critical role because this ability is the foundation of human creativity. Creation comes from the imagination. Having only desire is one thing; being able to imagine and implement that desire is another thing altogether. When we can picture clearly what we want, we can set our goals and know in which direction to go.

Vision Meditation is for drawing a desired state or goal as realistically as possible by using positive thoughts, emotions, and imagery. To begin, the entire energy system must be fully activated and the mind must achieve a state of relaxed concentration. This type of meditation helps us apply the things we have gained from training to our daily lives.

1. Sit in a half lotus position and straighten your back. Do Ji-gam and Dahn-mu for a while.

2. Once you feel the surrounding energy field, hold your hands over your head, without touching, and feel the flow of energy emanating from your brain.

3. As you feel the energy from your brain, spread your fingers apart and bring them in again to expand the feeling of the energy. Bring your hands closer and push them farther out from your head as you feel the force of the energy manifest as magnetic attraction and repulsion.

4. Let the movement of your hands, breath, and brain synchronize into one rhythm.

5. Imagine your body inflating and deflating like a large balloon with the rhythm of the breath.

6. Create a picture in your mind of what you want to be or the goal that you want to achieve.

7. Imagine in detail that your desire has already been achieved and give yourself self-acknowledgment and a self-assuring message.

8. Lower your hands to your knees or rest your cupped hands on your heels and keep meditating.

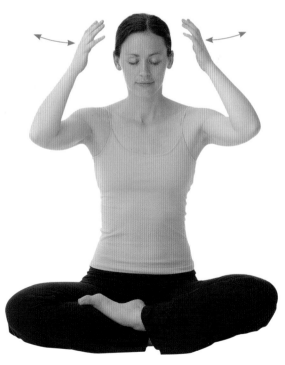

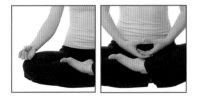

The Dahn Yoga Posture Chart

This chart provides an overview of all the postures in the book which you should refer to when planning what to practice in your daily routine.

MERIDIAN STRETCHING

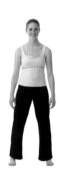

Basic Posture

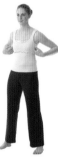

Body Bounce

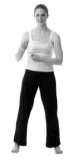

Upper Body Tapping

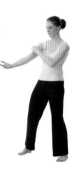

Whole Body Patting

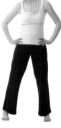

Neck Stretch

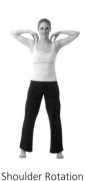

Shoulder Rotation

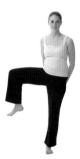

Standing Stretch

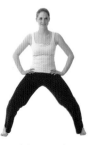

Hip Rotation

Pelvic Rotation

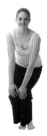

Knee Rotation

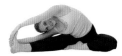
Side Stretch

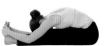
Sitting Forward Bend

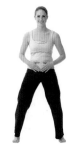
Straddle with Forward Bend

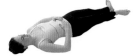
Toe Tapping

Rolling Back

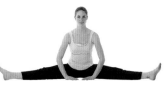
Abdominal Clapping   Intestine Exercise

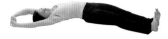
Whole Body Stretch

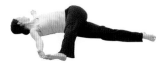
Crossing Leg to Fingers

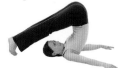
Lifting Legs over Head

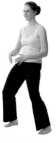
Upper Body Lift

JUNG-CHOONG BREATHING

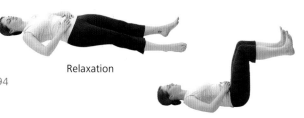

Relaxation

Accumulation

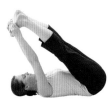

Circulation 1

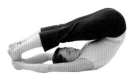

Circulation 2

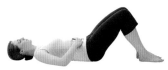

Relaxation and Accumulation

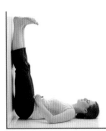

Legs Up the Wall
Accumulation

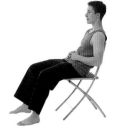

Accumulation in a Chair

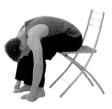

Circulation in a Chair

modifications

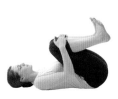

Accumulation

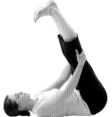

Circulation 1

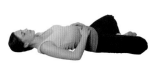

Relaxation and Accumulation

DAHNMUDO

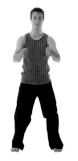

Waste-Hip Rotation

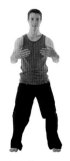

Chuk-ki Stance

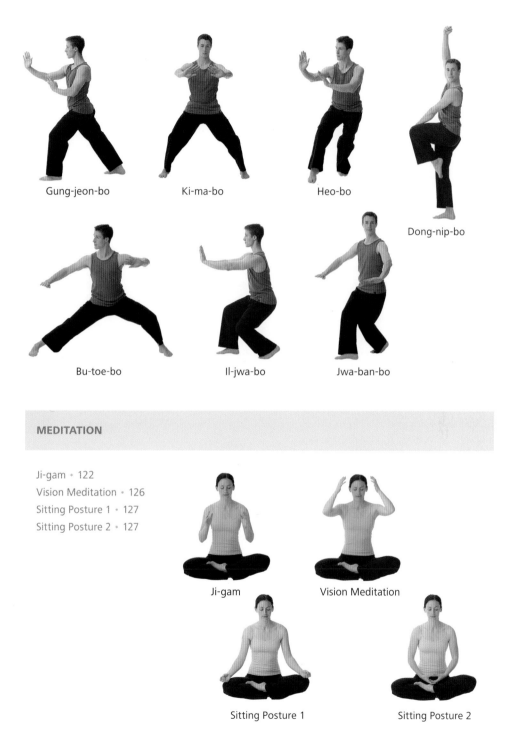

Gung-jeon-bo

Ki-ma-bo

Heo-bo

Dong-nip-bo

Bu-toe-bo

Il-jwa-bo

Jwa-ban-bo

MEDITATION

Ji-gam

Vision Meditation

Sitting Posture 1

Sitting Posture 2

Recommended Reading

BOOKS

Meridian Exercise for Self-Healing Book 1 & 2

Classified by Common Symptoms By Ilchi Lee

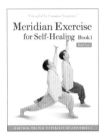

A systematic series of exercises that increase flexibility, balance, and strength of the body. These postures will stimulate and facilitate the natural flow of energy. Poses are explained in a detailed and friendly manner and are broken down into a step-by-step explanation.

Home Massage Therapy Book 1 & 2

Heal Yourself and Your Loved Ones
By Dahn Healer School

This series of Dahn healing techniques maximizes your body's healing capacity by stimulating relaxation points, meridians, and organs of the body. This book provides detailed illustrations that show a step-by-step guide to each healing technique.

Brain Respiration

Making Your Brain Creative, Peaceful, and Productive By Ilchi Lee
Explains the principles and methods of Brain Respiration, a mind-body training program that

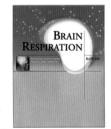

helps you obtain physical, mental, and spiritual health as you optimize brain function.

Human Technology

A Toolkit for Authentic Living By Ilchi Lee

A guidebook for personal self-mastery and fulfillment, this book encapsulates an enlightened way of thinking about ourselves, our fellow human beings, and all aspects of our life. A profound positive-thinking guide for self-improvement and personal contentment.

Healing Chakra

Light to awaken my soul By Ilchi Lee

This beautiful self-training package (book + CD) is designed to activate, balance, and integrate the individual chakras in order to create a harmonious and holistic chakra system.

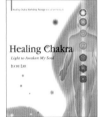

Dahnhak Kigong

Using the Body to Enlighten the Mind
By Ilchi Lee

A must-read for advanced practitioners and Kigong lovers. Develop gentle power, create serenity in movement, and achieve balance by reawakening the Ki-energy sensation. This book includes vivid color photos and fine illustrations, providing a step-by-step guide to each Kigong movement.

Healing Society

A Prescription for Global Enlightenment
By Ilchi Lee

Ilchi Lee's first book released in English, it reached #1 on Amazon.com within a month of publication. The author emphasizes that enlightenment is not just for a select few, but available to everyone. This book includes stories of the author's personal experiences during his quest to find the meaning of life.

SELF-TRAINING CDS

Brain Respiration Self-Training CD
Making Your Brain Creative, Peaceful, and Productive **By Ilchi Lee**

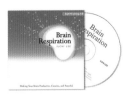

This self-training CD presents precise and concise instructions on all key phases of Brain Respiration, including energy sensitivity training and the five steps of Brain Respiration. All tracks are accompanied by meditative and stirring background music.

A Journey to You
By Arang Park
Ideal background music for meditation. This music CD is designed to deepen your meditation, nurture healing and renewal, and draw upon your innate inner wisdom.

VIDEOS AND DVDS

Dahn Yoga for Beginners (VHS/DVD)
Stretch Your Body, Expand Your Mind

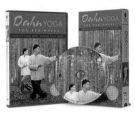

An easy-to-follow, step-by-step guide to the basic Dahn Yoga workout. Discover how to de-stress and relax through Dahn yoga practice, learn how to feel and utilize Ki (Chi) while developing inner peace and external strength.

If you are unable to order these products from your local book seller, you may order through www.amazon.com or www.bodynbrain.com.

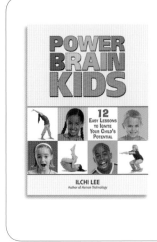

Power Brain Kids
12 Easy Lessons to Ignite Your Child's Potential

In this book you will find a child-appropriate and parent-friendly guide to Ilchi Lee's Brain Education (BE) method. Each lesson focuses on a particular mental ability, including concentration, creativity, memory, and emotional control. The colorful design and charming full-color photography will help to keep your child interested and involved with the lessons. Through the book, straight-A and struggling students alike will be challenged to apply their brains toward the creation of a genuinely happy and successful life.

Glossary

A

Abdominal Breathing See Dahn-jon Breathing.

Ah-moon An acupressure point located between the first and second vertebrae.

B

Baek-hoe An acupressure point located at the top of the head.

C

Chakra A Sanskrit word meaning a wheel or circle, it refers to any of the seven internal energy centers in the body.

Cham-jun-kye-kyung An ancient Korean scripture revealing 366 wisdoms that people can apply to everyday life.

Chest Breathing A breathing method designed to release tension through the loosening and relaxation of the chest.

Chi See Ki.

Chun-bu-kyung An ancient Korean scripture known as The Heavenly Code. It explains the trinity of Heaven, Earth, and Human.

Chun-ji-ki-woon Cosmic energy or the highest level of energy.

Chun-ji-ma-eum Cosmic mind or enlightened consciousness.

Conception meridian See Im-maek.

D

Dahn-jon Breathing A breathing method designed to take energy into the body and accumulate it in the lower Dahn-jon, an energy center in the lower abdomen.

Dahn-jon System The interrelated system of seven Dahn-jons (energy centers) in the body, which includes three internal Dahn-jons and four external Dahn-jons.

Dahn-jon An energy center in the body where energy (Ki) is accumulated. The word most often refers to the lower Dahn-jon located in the lower abdomen.

Dahn-mu A form of dancing that follows the natural flow of energy.

DahnMuDo A Korean non-combative, healing martial art based on Dahn principles.

Dahn Yoga A holistic health and mind-body training program that combines deep stretching exercises, meditative breathing techniques, and energy awareness training.

Dae-chu An accupressure point located right below the seventh cervical vertebrae.

Dahn The Korean word which means energy, vitality, and origin of life.

Dahn-joong An accupressure point located in the center of the slight indentation on the chest.

Dahnhak The original name of Dahn Yoga. It literally means "the study of life energy."

Dok-maek A major energy pathway that flows up the back of the body.

E

External Dahn-jons Energy centers located in the palms of both hands (see Jang-shim) and the soles of both feet (see Yong-chun).

G

Governing meridian See Dok-maek.

H

Hoe-eum An acupressure point located at the perineum.

I

Im-maek An energy pathway that flows down the front of the body.

In-dang An acupressure point, located between the eyebrows, which is also called "the Third Eye."

In-joong An acupressure point located in the center of the indentation between your nose and lips.

Internal Dahn-jons The three main energy centers located in the abdomen, chest, and head.

J

Jang-shim An acupressure point located at the center of the palm on each hand.

Ji-gam A meditative exercise to introduce the awareness of energy.

Jin-dong A healing phenomena resulting from stimulation of the energy system, which is characterized by mild to intense vibration of the body.

Jin-ki Unlimited energy which is received through pure cosmic awareness and accessed through deep mindful concentration of the breath.

Jun-jung An acupressure point located on the scalp, in between the hairline and the crown of the head.

Jung-Choong Breathing A breathing technique that combines sequential movements with focused breathing. This practice facilitates energy accumulation and proper energy circulation.

Jung-choong, Ki-jang, and Shin-myung One of the three principles of Dahn Yoga practice, which means, "Physical energy is filled, the energy body becomes strong, and spirituality is awakened."

Jung-ki Limited energy which is acquired from outside nourishment, such as through diet and respiration.

K

Ki-hae An acupressure point, located about 2 inches below the navel on the surface of the skin. It literally means "the sea of energy."

Ki The vital energy which circulates throughout the universe, the essence of every creation in the cosmos.

L

Lower Dahn-jon A major internal energy center located two inches below the navel and two inches inside the abdomen. It is associated with physical energy.

M

Meridian Stretching A system of exercise designed to open the meridian system of the body and to balance the energy. Also called "Do-in" exercise.

Meridian A pathway through which energy moves in the body.

Mi-gan An acupressure point located in the indention at the top of your nose.

Middle Dahn-jon A major internal energy center located in the middle of the chest. It is associated with mental and emotional energy.

Myung-hyun A healing phenomena which occurs as the body struggles to regain balance. It literally means "alternating brightness and darkness" and may include uncomfortable symptoms, such as dizziness, body aches, coughing, stuffy nose, etc.

Myung-moon An acupressure point located on the back, opposite the navel between the second and the third lumbar vertebrae.

R

Relaxed concentration The state of focusing on something while maintaining a relaxed body and mind.

S

Shim-ki-hyul-jung One of the three main principles of Dahn Yoga Practice, which literally means "where consciousness lies, energy flows, bringing blood and transforming the body." More simply stated, it means, "Where mind goes, energy follows."

Su-seung-hwa-gang One of the three main principles of Dahn Yoga, which means "water energy up, fire energy down."

T

Tae-yang A set of two acupressure points located on the sides of the head, one on each temple.

U

Un-ki-bo-hyung-gong A fundamental form of DahnMuDo consisting of seven sets.

Upper Dahn-jon A major internal energy center located just above and between the eyebrows in the center of the brain. It is associated with spiritual and intellectual energy.

V

Vision meditation A mediation technique for drawing out a desired goal or state of being as realistically as possible by using positive thoughts, emotions, and imagery.

W

Water Up, Fire Down *See* Su-seung-hwa-gang.

Won-ki Limited energy which is inherited through genetic information from the parents.

Y

Yong-chun An acupressure point located on the sole of each foot. It is approximately in the center of the foot, and just below the ball.

Index

Dahn Yoga Centers

USA

ARIZONA

Ahwatukee
480-783-4885(T) / 4886(F)

Chandler
480-857-9642(T) / 9644(F)

East Mesa
480-924-9642(T) / 9643(F)

Gilbert
480-632-9642(T) / 9643(F)

Glendale
602-439-9642(T) / 9645(F)

Scottsdale
480-391-8916(T) / 8917(F)

Sedona
928-282-3600(T) / 1854(F)

Tempe
480-345-9642(T) / 9646(F)

NORTHERN CALIFORNIA

Fremont
510-979-1130(T) / 0240(F)

Mt. View
650-960-1717(T) / 1711(F)

San Mateo
650-577-0321(T) / 1033(F)

Santa Clara
408-241-0328(T) / 1289(F)

SOUTHERN CALIFORNIA

Anaheim Hills
714-283-0046(T) / 0048(F)

Beverly Hills
310-788-9642(T) / 9641(F)

Brea
714-990-3550(T) / 2250(F)

SUN Institute LA Campus
714-992-5126(T) / 5102(F)

Encinitas
760-436-0800(T) / 0318(F)

Fullerton
714-994-1306, 670-2050(T)
/ 670-2028(F)

Garden Grove
714-537-3499(T) / 3622(F)

Glendale
818-265-9356(T) / 9354(F)

Irvine
714-669-8330(T) / 8328(F)

Mission Viejo
949-583-9133(T) / 9139(F)

Oak Park
818-889-9642(T) / 9643(F)

Oceanside
760-758-0906(T) / 0946(F)

Olympic
213-381-3893(T) / 3892(F)

Rolling Hills
310-265-9642(T) / 9635(F)

Torrance
310-791-0301(T) / 0365(F)

Valencia
661-263-9777(T) / 9457(F)

Valley
818-343-6960(T) / 8922(F)

COLORADO

Aurora
303-400-5323(T) / 5157(F)

Boulder
720-565-0609(T) / 0610(F)

Buckley
303-369-6135(T) / 6138(F)

Denver
303-694-2717(T) / 3717(F)

Kipling
303-948-5500(T) / 5700(F)

Lakewood
303-716-2700(T) / 9642(F)

Westminster
303-456-7670(T) / 7688(F)

CONNECTICUT

Avon
860-676-9642(T) /
409-2141(F)

DISTRICT OF COLUMBIA

Georgetown
202-298-3246(T) / 7212(F)

Van Ness
202-237-9642(T)

Washington, DC
202-393-2440(T) / 2441(F)

GEORGIA

Atlanta (Midtown)
404-541-0966(T)

Buckhead
404-252-1881(T) / 1880(F)

Duluth
678-475-0405(T) / 0490(F)

Marietta
770-971-1171(T) / 1174(F)

Peachtree Buckhead
404-841-9995(T) / 9964

Roswell
770-643-2220(T) / 2820(F)

Sandy Spring
404-497-0202(T) / 0203(F)
Vinings
770-435-4335(T) / 4316
HAWAII
Aiea
808-486-9642(T) /
488-3389(F)
Honolulu
808-942-0003(T) /
943-0523(F)
ILLINOIS
Buffalo Grove
847-808-9642(T) /
279-1751(F)
Chicago
773-539-4467(T) / 4468(F)
Crystal Lake
815-356-0727(T) / 0726(F)
Forest Park
708-771-9642(T) / 4061(F)
Glenview
847-998-1377(T) / 1376(F)
Lake View Lincoln Park
773-755-9566(T) / 9564(F)
Libertyville
847-362-2724(T) / 2721(F)
Michigan
312-263-9642(T) / 9365(F)
Naperville
630-505-0809(T) / 0805(F)
Orland Park
708-226-0245(T) / 0246(F)
Palatine
847-358-7017 / 7027(F)
Schaumburg
847-882-6980(T) / 6552(F)
St. Charles
630-443-9642(T) / 0670(F)
Westmont
630-230-0365(T) / 0368(F)

MARYLAND
Beltsville
301-595-2056(T) / 7155(F)
Bethesda
301-907-6520(T) / 6521(F)
College Park
301-699-9642(T) / 9644(F)
Gaithersburg
301-330-4861(T) / 4862(F)
Rockville
301-424-9033(T) / 9034(F)
MASSACHUSETTS
Andover
978-475-1116(T)
Arlington
781-648-9642(T) / 9643(F)
Beacon Hill
617-742-9642(T) / 9632(F)
Belmont
617-484-9642(T)
Brookline
617-264-4851(T) / 4852(F)
Copley
617-262-9642(T) / 9643(F)
Boston, MA 02118
Havard
617-576-9642(T) / 9643(F)
Jamaica Plain
617-983-9642(T) / 9643(F)
Melrose
781-979-0066(T) / 0060
Newton
617-964-8333(T) / 3005(F)
Somerville
617-623-3246(T) /
764-1778(F)
MICHIGAN
Utica
586-739-9642(T) / 8064(F)
West Bloomfield
248-855-0314(T) / 0214(F)

NEVADA
Henderson
702-432-0008(T) /
870-1112(F)
Las Vegas
702-256-6778(T) / 0385(F)
NEW JERSEY
CGI BR
201-784-5575(T) / 2466(F)
Hoboken
201-795-1777(T)
Madison
973-377-4567(T)
Montvale BR
201-476-0002(T)
Oradell
201-225-9000(T) / 0086(F)
Ridgefield
201-941-8622(T) / 1192(F)
Sun Institute NJ Campus
201-225-9000(T) / 0086(F)
Westfield
908-301-9642(T) / 9094(F)
West Orange
973-731-1550(T) / 1552(F)
Wyckoff
201-444-6020(T)
NEW MEXICO
Albuquerque
505-797-2211(T) / 2895(F)
Cottonwood
505-792-5111(T) / 3444(F)
Nob Hill
505-262-2211(T) / 2212(F)
Santa Fe
505-820-2211(T) /
982-8670(F)
NEW YORK
Astoria
718-626-0560(T) / 0561(F)

Bay Ridge
718-765-0099(T) / 0089(F)

Bedford BR
914-242-8800(T) / 3898(F)

Bronx
718-892-1100(T) / 8100(F)

Brooklyn Heights
718-254-8833(T) / 8855(F)

East Meadow
516-227-0101(T) / 5342(F)

Flushing
718-762-6373(T) /
539-7286(F)

Forest Hills
718-261-5588(T) / 2252(F)

Franklin Square
516-481-2526(T) / 2534(F)

Great Neck
516-487-8406(T) / 8196(F)

Manhattan
212-725-3262(T) /
683-2571(F)

Manhattan BR
212-935-5777(T) /
906-0067(F)

Massapequa
516-795-0456(T) / 0282(F)

New City BR
845-638-2100(T) /
634-9500(F)

Park East BR
212-249-0077(T) / 0074(F)

Smithtown
631-724-0686(T) / 0796(F)

Syosset
516-364-3413(T) / 4654(F)

Union Square BR
212-691-7799(T) / 7798(F)

Westchester BR
914-713-1333(T) / 1359(F)

Ashland
541-552-1040(T) / 1014(F)

Beaverton
503-521-9793(T) / 9795(F)

Eugene
541-686-0207(T) / 0209(F)

Medford
541-770-9191(T) / 9561(F)

Portland
503-248-2104(T) / 2094(F)

West Linn
503-657-3673(T) / 3638(F)

Austin
512-347-7575(T) / 7577(F)

Belt Line
972-687-0011(T) / 0094(F)

Champion
281-440-6160(T) / 6366(F)

Clear Lake
281-480-9642(T) / 9643(F)

Copperfield
832-237-9642(T) / 9641(F)

Eldridge
281-497-9642(T) / 9643(F)

Katy
281-492-7000(T) / 7987(F)

Kingwood
281-540-3246(T) / 3247(F)

Memorial
713-464-7012(T) / 7085(F)

Missouri City
281-261-9979(T) / 9994(F)

River Oaks
713-529-9642(T) / 9646(F)

Sugar Land
281-242-3246(T) / 3258(F)

Voss
832-251-9642(T) / 9644(F)

West Park
713-664-3246(T) / 3245(F)

Alexandria
703-684-7717(T) / 7718(F)

Burke
703-866-9642(T) / 9643(F)

Centreville
703-266-5363(T) / 5364(F)

Crystal City
703-413-6942(T) / 9643(F)

Leesburg
703-779-6942(T) / 0630(F)

Mclean
703-442-3246

Vienna
703-242-9373(T) / 9374(F)

Ballinger
206-366-1122, 2738(T) /
2739(F)

Bellevue
425-373-9959(T) /
378-3439(F)

Harbor Steps
206-223-9642(T) / 9645(F)

Kirkland
425-893-9642(T) / 827-
0200(F)

Mill Creek
425-357-6060(T)

Sammamish
425-836-1113(T) / 1799(F)

Tacoma
253-566-9642(T) / 9644(F)

U.W.
206-524-7166(T) / 7199(F)

CANADA

ALBERTA
Shawnessy
403-256-4044(T)
BRITISH COLUMBIA
Kitsilano
604-714-0074(T) / 0084(F)
Vancouver
604-988-7499(T) / 7496(F)
ONTARIO
Burlington
905-681-7215(T) / 1298(F)
Dream Crest
905-858-0036(T)
Hampton Park
613-761-8000(T)
Mississauga
905-281-3467(T) / 0700(F)
North York
416-630-3157(T) / 6083(F)
Thornhill
905-763-0100(T) / 0500(F)
QUEBEC
Brossard
450-656-1700(T)
Laval
450-669-3246(T)
Montreal
514-845-4888(T)

SOUTH AMERICA

BRAZIL
São Paulo
55-11-223-6460(T)

UNITED KINGDOM

BRIGHTON
Brighton HSP Centre
44-1273-357-559(T)
LONDON
Battersea
44-208-222-8542(T)
Hammersmith
44-208-222-8542(T)
Putney
44-208-780-2555(T)
SURREY
Epsom
44-1372-743-991(T)
Surbiton
44-208-339 3776(T)
Walton-on-Thames
44-1932-259-759(T)

Visit www.hspholistic.com

ASIA

JAPAN
Visit www.DahnHak.co.jp
KOREA
Visit www.DahnWorld.com

*For more information
visit www.dahnyoga.com
call 1-877-HSP-YOGA*

ACKNOWLEDGEMENTS
*Healing Society would like
to extend special thanks to:*

Models
Erin Carter
Aaron Daniels
Stephanie Jasieniecki

Photographs
Paul Markow
Myungsoon Kim

Translation
JooRi Jun
Daniel T. Graham

Design
Ji-in Kim
Michele Blink

Editing
Nicole Dean
Catherine Rourke

Illustrations
Junghyun Sohn